ESSENTIALS

of DIAGNOSIS
& TREATMENT
in CARDIOLOGY

a LANGE medical book

ESSENTIALS
of DIAGNOSIS
& TREATMENT
in CARDIOLOGY

Michael H. Crawford, MD
Professor of Medicine
Associate Chief of Cardiology for Clinical Programs
University of California, San Francisco

Komandoor Srivathson, MD
Instructor in Medicine
Mayo Medical School
Rochester, Minnesota

Lange Medical Books/McGraw-Hill
Medical Publishing Division

New York   Chicago   San Francisco   Lisbon   London   Madrid   Mexico City
Milan   New Delhi   San Juan   Seoul   Singapore   Sydney   Toronto

The **McGraw·Hill** Companies

Essentials of Diagnosis & Treatment in Cardiology

2   3   4   5   6   7   8   9   0   DOCDOC   0   9   8   7   6   5   4

ISBN: 0-07-142321-4
ISSN: 1547-2876

NOTICE

Medicine is an ever-changing science. As new research and clinical experience broaden our knowledge, changes in treatment and drug therapy are
required. The authors and the publisher of this work have checked with
sources believed to be reliable in their efforts to provide information that is
complete and generally in accord with the standards accepted at the time of
publication. However, in view of the possibility of human error or changes
in medical sciences, neither the authors nor the publisher nor any other party
who has been involved in the preparation or publication of this work warrants
that the information contained herein is in every respect accurate or complete,
and they disclaim all responsibility for any errors or omissions or for the
results obtained from use of the information contained in this work. Readers
are encouraged to confirm the information contained herein with other
sources. For example and in particular, readers are advised to check the prod-
uct information sheet included in the package of each drug they plan to
administer to be certain that the information contained in this work is accurate and that changes have not been made in the recommended dose or in the
contraindications for administration. This recommendation is of particular
importance in connection with new or infrequently used drugs.

This book was set in Times Roman by International Typesetting
    and Composition.
The editors were Isabel Nogueira, Harriet Lebowitz, and Peter J. Boyle.
The production supervisor was Phil Galea.
The cover designer was Elizabeth Pisacreta.
The index was prepared by Patricia Perrier.
RR Donnelley was printer and binder.

This book is printed on acid-free paper.

Contents

Preface

This book is intended as a support and companion volume to *Current Diagnosis & Treatment in Cardiology,* now in its second edition and widely used. It is arranged in ten sections with main subject titles in alphabetical order for easy retrieval "on the job," as it were—making rounds, responding to clinical calls—as well as preparing for classroom participation or Board examinations. Coverage is offered not only of the more common heart diseases but also of some disorders of occasional or exotic interest such as tako-tsubo cardiomyopathy.

What the reader will find in these pages represents the critical details of diagnosis—including differential diagnosis—and treatment of clinical cardiologic entities, including arrhythmias, vascular diseases, congenital disorders, and even some systemic and neuromuscular diseases, drug toxicities, and metabolic and endocrine disorders that may involve the cardiovascular system. Medical education and enhanced patient care are the goals we aspire to in offering this book for distribution.

Michael H. Crawford, MD
Komandoor Srivathson, MD

January 2004

1

Ischemic Heart Disease

Angina Pectoris, Unstable

- ■ Essentials of Diagnosis
  - New or worsening symptoms (angina, pulmonary edema) or signs (electrocardiographic [ECG] changes) of myocardial ischemia
  - Absence or mild elevation of cardiac enzymes (creatinine kinase and its MB fraction or troponin I or T) without prolonged ST-segment elevation on ECG
  - Unstable angina and non-ST elevation myocardial infarction are closely related in pathogenesis and clinical presentation and are often considered one entity

- ■ Differential Diagnosis
  - Stable angina pectoris
  - Variant angina
  - Myocardial infarction
  - Aortic dissection
  - Acute myopericarditis
  - Acute pulmonary embolism
  - Esophageal reflux
  - Cholecystitis
  - Peptic ulcer disease
  - Cervical radiculopathy
  - Costochondritis
  - Pneumothorax

- ■ Treatment
  - Hospitalization with ECG monitoring, bed rest, oxygen
  - Elimination of aggravating factors, such as hypertension, dysrhythmias, anemia, heart failure, thyrotoxicosis
  - Aspirin 162 mg
  - Nitrates, usually intravenous (IV) or cutaneous, for pain
  - Heparin, either unfractionated or low molecular weight
  - Beta-blockers for continued pain
  - Calcium channel blockers when beta-blockers are contraindicated or pain is refractory
  - Clopidogrel for patients who cannot take aspirin or before angioplasty in high-risk patients
  - Platelet glycoprotein IIb/IIIa inhibitors for high-risk patients, especially if percutaneous revascularization is planned
  - Revascularization:
    Percutaneous coronary intervention early for high-risk patients
    Coronary artery bypass graft surgery for high-risk patients in whom angioplasty is not feasible or unsuccessful
  - Intra-aortic balloon counterpulsation to stabilize hemodynamically unstable patients for catheterization or surgery

- ■ Pearl

In patients with unstable chest pain syndromes and no specific diagnosis, noninvasive stress testing is contraindicated until patients are pain free without IV medications for 24–48 hours.

Reference

TACTICS-TIMI 18 investigators: Comparison of early invasive and conservative strategies in patients with unstable coronary syndromes treated with the glycoprotein IIb/IIIa inhibitor tirofiban. N Engl J Med 2001;344:1879.

Cardiac Allograft Vasculopathy

- **Essentials of Diagnosis**
  - Incidence is 20–50% at 5 years
  - It is the main cause of late post-transplant deaths and is the main factor limiting long-term survival
  - Angina pectoris is rare because of allograft denervation
  - Myocardial infarction, impaired left ventricular function with heart failure, arrhythmias, and sudden death may occur
  - Recipient characteristics (eg, hypertension, hyperlipidemia, insulin resistance, and cytomegalovirus infection) and donor characteristics (eg, preexisting coronary disease, donor ischemic time) may play a role
  - Noninvasive tests (except perhaps dobutamine stress echocardiography) are not useful in assessing this disease

- **Differential Diagnosis**
  - Acute rejection
  - Cytomegalovirus infection

- **Prevention & Treatment**
  - Diltiazem and lipid-lowering agents are useful for prevention
  - Risk factor modification may help in prevention
  - Percutaneous coronary intervention may be useful in some cases
  - Retransplantation is a choice for diffuse vasculopathy, but is associated with a low survival rate

- **Pearl**

A negative noninvasive test does not exclude allograft vasculopathy.

Reference

Weis M: Cardiac allograft vasculopathy: Prevention and treatment options. Transplant Proc 2002;34:1847.

Cardiac Syndrome X (Microvascular Angina Pectoris)

- ■ Essentials of Diagnosis
  - Typical angina pectoris
  - Positive stress test for myocardial ischemia, especially exercise ECG or stress myocardial perfusion abnormalities
  - Normal or near normal epicardial coronary arteries
  - Usually women (75%); many also have neuropsychological symptoms
  - No evidence of coronary spasm on ambulatory ECG monitoring or coronary angiography

- ■ Differential Diagnosis
  - Variant angina pectoris
  - Missed coronary artery lesions because of inadequate angiography
  - Other causes of chest pain with a false-positive stress test
  - Neuropsychiatric disorder

- ■ Treatment
  - Reassurance; prognosis is good
  - Calcium channel blockers
  - Nitrates and beta-blockers for selected patients
  - Aminophylline for selected patients
  - Imipramine for refractory cases
  - Spinal cord stimulation in selected cases

- ■ Pearl

In patients with angina pectoris and normal coronary arteries, long-term survival is good regardless of whether stress testing is positive.

Reference

Buus NH et al: Reduced vasodilator capacity in syndrome X related to structure and function of resistance arteries. Am J Cardiol 1999;83:149.

Coronary Artery Disease, Symptomatic Non-Revascularizable

- ■ **Essentials of Diagnosis**
  - • Persistent angina pectoris despite maximally tolerated doses of nitrates, beta-blockers, and calcium channel blockers
  - • Diffuse coronary atherosclerosis not amenable to revascularization
  - • Relatively normal left ventricular function, which excludes heart transplantation

- ■ **Differential Diagnosis**
  - • Precipitating or aggravating conditions such as hypertension, anemia, thyrotoxicosis
  - • Less than maximal medical therapy
  - • Second opinion on lack of feasibility of revascularization

- ■ **Treatment**
  - • Spinal cord stimulation
  - • Enhanced external counterpulsation
  - • Transmyocardial laser revascularization
  - • Gene therapy locally, such as vascular endothelial growth factor, is under investigation

- ■ **Pearl**

Angiotensin-converting enzyme inhibitors are not antianginal. If their use is solely prophylactic and they are lowering the blood pressure excessively or to the extent that maximal doses of true antianginal drugs cannot be administered, their dosage should be decreased or they should be eliminated.

Reference

Arora RR et al. The multicenter study of enhanced external counterpulsation (MUST-EECP): Effect of EECP on exercise-induced myocardial ischemia and angina episodes. J Am Coll Cardiol 1999;33:1833.

Hibernating & Stunned Myocardium

- **Essentials of Diagnosis**
  - Stunned: prolonged myocardial contractile dysfunction after a brief period of absent or reduced blood flow
  - Hibernating: myocardial contractile dysfunction associated with reduced blood flow that reverses with revascularization
  - Imaging evidence of myocardial viability: delayed thallium uptake, wall motion response to dobutamine infusion, metabolic activity on positron emission tomography scan

- **Differential Diagnosis**
  - Stunned: acute ischemia with compromised blood flow
  - Hibernating: infarcted myocardium

- **Treatment**
  - Stunned: calcium channel blockers, angiotensin-converting enzyme inhibitors, positive inotropic agents, circulatory support (see cardiogenic shock)
  - Hibernating: coronary artery revascularization

- **Pearl**

Noninvasive imaging studies are not 100% accurate for predicting viable, hibernating myocardium. Thus, in patients with ischemic left ventricular dysfunction, revascularization is appropriate in suitable patients despite a negative viability study.

Reference

Schinkel AF et al: Dobutamine-induced contractile reserve in stunned, hibernating, and scarred myocardium in patients with ischemic cardiomyopathy. J Nucl Med 2003;44:127.

In-Stent Restenosis

- **Essentials of Diagnosis**
  - Focal intimal proliferation inside the stent or at the edges, resulting in restenosis
  - Diffuse intimal proliferation and restenosis in the stent
  - Original stented lesion was long or had a small lumen diameter
  - Diabetic patients have a higher occurrence
  - Recurrent angina or detection on routine stress tests, confirmed at angiography

- **Differential Diagnosis**
  - Symptoms early after stenting (<1 month) usually mean in-stent thrombosis
  - Symptoms late after stenting (>9 months) usually mean progressive disease in non-stented segments
  - Other causes of chest pain or positive stress tests may be found

- **Treatment**
  - Balloon angioplasty, especially for focal lesions
  - Repeat stenting, especially with drug-eluting stents
  - Catheter-delivered radiation (brachytherapy) usually as an adjunct to repeat angioplasty or stenting

- **Pearl**

Chest pain in the first 24–49 hours following percutaneous coronary interventions is common and usually not due to in-stent thrombosis. The resting ECG is the best triage tool. Ischemic changes suggest thrombosis. An ECG done during balloon inflation is useful as a comparison. Also, radionuclide myocardial perfusion imaging may be falsely positive within 1–3 months of successful angioplasty. Symptoms in this period usually necessitate repeat catheterization.

Reference

McPherson JA et al: Angiographic findings in patients undergoing catheterization for recurrent symptoms within 30 days of successful coronary intervention. Am J Cardiol 1999;84:589.

Ischemic Heart Disease, Chronic

- **Essentials of Diagnosis**
  - Typical exertional angina pectoris or its equivalents
  - Objective evidence of myocardial ischemia by ECG, myocardial imaging, or myocardial perfusion scanning
  - Likely occlusive coronary artery disease because of history and objective evidence of prior myocardial infarction
  - Known coronary artery disease shown by coronary angiography

- **Differential Diagnosis**
  - Other causes of chest pain (eg, esophageal reflux, costochondritis)
  - False-positive evidence of ischemia (eg, cardiomyopathy, technical shortcomings of tests)
  - Cholecystitis
  - Peptic ulcer disease
  - Cervical radiculopathy

- **Treatment**
  - Treat reversible risk factors for coronary artery disease such as smoking, hypertension, hypercholesterolemia, hyperglycemia, inflammation
  - Eliminate factors that aggravate myocardial oxygen supply/demand imbalance, such as tachyarrhythmias, thyrotoxicosis, anemia, hypoxia, heart failure, catecholamine analogues (eg, bronchodilators)
  - Pharmacologic therapy—sublingual nitroglycerin for acute angina episodes
  - Prophylactic therapy—aspirin, long-acting nitrates, beta-blockers, calcium blockers
  - Revascularization for persistently symptomatic patients:
    Percutaneous coronary intervention (angioplasty, stenting) for suitable coronary anatomy
    Coronary artery bypass graft surgery favored for left main disease and 2- or 3-vessel disease with involvement of the left anterior descending coronary artery, reduced left ventricular function, or diabetes

- **Pearl**

Some patients with chronic ischemic heart disease have symptoms such as dyspnea or profound weakness and diaphoresis on exertion (angina equivalents) but no chest pain.

Reference

Thadani U: Management of stable angina pectoris. Prog Cardiovasc Dis 1999;14:349.

Left Ventricular Aneurysm

- ### Essentials of Diagnosis
  - True aneurysm: echocardiographic evidence of thinned, scarred myocardium that deforms the diastolic silhouette of the left ventricle with systolic akinesis or dyskinesis
  - False aneurysm: echocardiographic evidence of a thin-walled sac communicating with an infarcted segment of the left ventricle by a narrow neck. Systolic expansion of the sac is often observed. Color flow imaging shows flow in and out of the sac.

- ### Differential Diagnosis
  - Akinetic or dyskinetic segments without diastolic deformity
  - Pericardial cyst or loculated effusion

- ### Treatment
  - True aneurysm; treat complications:
    Chronic anticoagulation to prevent thrombus formation
    Severe heart failure may benefit from aneurysmectomy
    Intractable arrhythmias may benefit from aneurysmectomy
  - Pseudoaneurysm: surgical correction to prevent rupture

- ### Pearl
True aneurysms rarely rupture, so routine surgical correction is not recommended.

Reference
Pasini S et al: Early and late results after surgical therapy of postinfarction left ventricular aneurysm. J Cardiovasc Surg 1998;39:209.

Left Ventricular Free Wall Rupture, Acute

- ■ Essentials of Diagnosis
  - Sudden marked bradycardia and hypotension up to 2 weeks after acute myocardial infarction
  - Cardiac arrest with electromechanical dissociation
  - Acute cardiac tamponade—elevated jugular venous pressure and hypotension

- ■ Differential Diagnosis
  - Acute ventricular septal rupture
  - Acute mitral regurgitation
  - Massive myocardial infarction
  - Arrhythmic cardiac arrest

- ■ Treatment
  - Immediate pericardiocentesis followed by emergency corrective surgery
  - Intra-aortic balloon counterpulsation to stabilize the patient for cardiac catheterization, if feasible
  - Percutaneous cardiopulmonary bypass in preparation for surgery

- ■ Pearl

Despite the hole in the left ventricle, a murmur is rarely heard in acute myocardial rupture. Subacute rupture may present as pericarditis.

Reference

Flajsig I: Surgical treatment of left ventricular free wall rupture after myocardial infarction: Case series. Croat Med J 2002;43:643.

Myocardial Infarction, Acute Non–ST-Segment Elevation

- ■ Essentials of Diagnosis
  - New or worsening angina pectoris or its equivalents
  - ST-wave depression or T-wave inversion (less specific) on ECG in 2 or more contiguous leads
  - Positive biologic markers for myocardial injury (ie, troponin or creatine kinase–MB)

- ■ Differential Diagnosis
  - Stable angina pectoris
  - Variant angina
  - Unstable angina
  - Aortic dissection
  - Acute myopericarditis
  - Acute pulmonary embolism
  - Esophageal reflux
  - Cholecystitis
  - Peptic ulcer disease
  - Cervical radiculopathy
  - Costochondritis
  - Pneumothorax

- ■ Treatment
  - General: Hospitalization with ECG monitoring, bed rest, and an IV line. Oxygen. Aspirin 162 mg. Pain relief with sublingual nitroglycerin followed by IV morphine sulfate
  - Specific pharmacologic therapy:
    Beta-blockers IV followed by oral unfractionated heparin or low-molecular-weight heparin; clopidogrel for aspirin-sensitive patients or those likely to have percutaneous revascularization
    Calcium channel blockers for refractory symptoms
    Platelet glycoprotein IIb/IIIa inhibitors
  - Revascularization—early coronary angiography is preferred, when feasible, with angioplasty or surgical revascularization as indicated
  - Intra-aortic balloon counterpulsation to stabilize hemodynamically unstable patients for catheterization or surgery

- ■ Pearl

  Non–ST-segment elevation myocardial infarction has the same pathophysiology and treatment as unstable angina. The only difference is that biologic markers are positive in the former, but not in the latter.

Reference

Wallentin L et al: Outcome at 1 year after an invasive compared with a non-invasive strategy in unstable coronary-artery disease: The FRISC II invasive randomized trial. FRISC II Investigators. Fast Revascularization During Instability in Coronary Artery Disease. Lancet 2000;356:9.

Myocardial Infarction, Acute ST Elevation

- ■ Essentials of Diagnosis
  - Evidence of myocardial injury
  - Elevated marker protein such as troponin
  - Evidence of acute myocardial ischemia
  - Clinical symptoms and signs
  - Characteristic ECG changes
  - Cardiac imaging

- ■ Differential Diagnosis
  - Stable angina pectoris
  - Variant angina
  - Unstable angina
  - Aortic dissection
  - Acute myopericarditis
  - Acute pulmonary embolism
  - Esophageal reflux
  - Cholecystitis
  - Peptic ulcer disease
  - Cervical radiculopathy
  - Costochondritis
  - Pneumothorax

- ■ Treatment
  - Immediate revascularization by percutaneous coronary intervention if it can be accomplished within 60 minutes, otherwise use IV thrombolytic therapy
  - Hospitalization with cardiac monitoring, IV access, bed rest, and oxygen
  - Aspirin 162 mg, or clopidogrel if patient is aspirin sensitive
  - Unfractionated heparin
  - Beta-blockers IV and then orally
  - Morphine sulfate for pain
  - Sublingual followed by IV nitroglycerin for pain
  - Angiotensin-converting enzyme inhibitors if blood pressure allows
  - Intra-aortic balloon counterpulsation to stabilize hemodynamically unstable patients for catheterization or surgery

- ■ Pearl

Cholesterol-lowering therapy should be started before discharge regardless of the cholesterol level, which is often paradoxically low for up to 3 months after acute myocardial infarction.

Reference

Zijlstra F et al: Clinical characteristics and outcome of patients with early (<2 h), intermediate (2–4 h) and late (>4 h) presentation treated by primary coronary angioplasty or thrombolytic therapy for acute myocardial infarction. Eur Heart J 2002;23:550.

Myocardial Infarction, Right Ventricular

■ **Essentials of Diagnosis**

- Symptoms consistent with acute myocardial infarction
- ECG changes of acute inferior or posterior ST-segment elevation myocardial infarction with ST elevation in V3R or V4R
- Elevated cardiac biomarkers
- Echocardiographic evidence of right ventricular wall motion abnormalities
- Hypotension and jugular venous distortion with clear lung fields are commonly observed
- In the setting of acute inferoposterior myocardial infarction, a mean right atrial to pulmonary wedge pressure ratio of 0.8 or higher

■ **Differential Diagnosis**

- Hypotension from other causes with inferoposterior myocardial infarction
- Pericarditis
- Pulmonary embolus
- Aortic dissection

■ **Treatment**

- Immediate coronary reperfusion
- IV fluids if left atrial pressure is low
- IV positive inotropic agents to maintain blood pressure
- Avoid diuretics and vasodilators
- Other treatment similar to that for acute ST-elevation myocardial infarction

■ **Pearl**

Fluid resuscitation used to be the mainstay of therapy, but often did not maintain blood pressure and caused peripheral and pulmonary edema. If initial fluid boluses do not raise the blood pressure, employ IV pressors early.

Reference

Kosuge M et al: New electrocardiographic criteria for predicting the site of coronary artery occlusion in inferior wall acute myocardial infarction. Am J Cardiol 1998;82:1318.

Myocardial Infarction with Normal Coronary Arteries, Acute

- **Essentials of Diagnosis**
  - Acute myocardial infarction documented
  - Normal or near normal coronary angiography

- **Differential Diagnosis & Causes**
  - Rupture of a minimal (<50% diameter narrowing) plaque with thrombus formation and subsequent dissolution
  - Cocaine or methamphetamine use
  - Spontaneous coronary vasospasm
  - Myocarditis
  - Coagulopathies or hyperviscosity syndromes
  - Coronary embolism, usually from left-heart chambers
  - Arteritis
  - Trauma

- **Treatment**
  - Thrombolysis for suspected thrombosis or embolism
  - Nitrates or calcium channel blockers to relieve spasm
  - Specific therapy for or elimination of precipitating factors
  - Secondary prevention measures as appropriate (eg, smoking cessation)

- **Pearl**

About 10% of patients with acute myocardial infarction have normal or minimal-lesion coronary arteries. This presentation is most common in young (age <40 years) smokers.

Reference

Sarda L et al: Myocarditis in patients with clinical presentation of myocardial infarction and normal coronary angiograms. J Am Coll Cardiol 2001;37:786.

Myocardial Ischemia, Asymptomatic

- ■ Essentials of Diagnosis
  - • Objective evidence of myocardial ischemia is present in the absence of angina pectoris or its equivalent
  - • Most patients have underlying coronary artery disease
  - • Ambulatory ECG monitoring shows ischemic ST transients during normal activities, or a positive stress test documents ischemia

- ■ Differential Diagnosis
  - • False-positive ECG or cardiac imaging studies
  - • Variant or vasospastic angina with atypical symptoms
  - • Defective pain sensation in diabetic patients with coronary artery disease

- ■ Treatment
  - • Beta-blockers are the mainstay of therapy because most episodes are associated with increased myocardial oxygen demand
  - • Nitrates and calcium channel blockers are less effective
  - • Revascularization is useful in selected patients
  - • Control any underlying atherosclerosis (ie, cholesterol lowering)

- ■ Pearl

Asymptomatic myocardial ischemia would be of no consequence if it were not associated with adverse clinical outcomes.

Reference

Pepine CJ et al: Relation between clinical, angiographic and ischemic findings at baseline and ischemia-related adverse outcomes at 1 year in the Asymptomatic Cardiac Ischemic Pilot Study. J Am Coll Cardiol 1997;29:1483.

Variant or Prinzmetal Angina

- **Essentials of Diagnosis**
  - Resting chest pain is typical of myocardial ischemia but does not occur with exercise
  - ECG exhibits transient ST-segment elevation
  - Pain and ECG changes resolve spontaneously or after nitroglycerin administration
  - Coronary angiography demonstrates focal arterial spasm

- **Differential Diagnosis**
  - Unstable chronic ischemic heart disease
  - Myocardial infarction
  - Pericarditis
  - ECG mimics early repolarization

- **Treatment**
  - Sublingual nitroglycerin for acute attacks
  - Long-acting nitrates
  - Calcium channel blockers
  - Avoid beta-blockers unless required for concomitant coronary atherosclerosis
  - Percutaneous or surgical revascularization is rarely successful

- **Pearl**

Persistent coronary artery spasm can lead to acute myocardial infarction, so variant angina is considered inherently unstable.

Reference

Sueda S et al: Limitations of medical therapy in patients with pure coronary spastic angina. Chest 2003;123:380.

Ventricular Septal Rupture, Acute

- **Essentials of Diagnosis**
  - New pansystolic murmur days after an acute myocardial infarction
  - Sudden hypotension or heart failure post myocardial infarction
  - Echocardiographic evidence of a ventricular septal defect

- **Differential Diagnosis**
  - Hypotension or heart failure with acute myocardial infarction for other reasons
  - Acute mitral regurgitation due to papillary muscle rupture or dysfunction
  - Cardiac rupture with pseudoaneurysm formation

- **Treatment**
  - Diuresis for heart failure
  - Pressor support for hypotension
  - IV sodium nitroprusside if blood pressure allows; intra-aortic balloon counterpulsation to stabilize the patient
  - Corrective surgery to substantially reduce mortality

- **Pearl**

Patients with acute ventricular septal rupture can often be distinguished from those with acute mitral regurgitation (although both present with heart failure and new pansystolic murmurs) because the latter usually have profound pulmonary edema.

Reference

Madsen JC, Daggett WM Jr: Repair of postinfarction ventricular septal defects. Semin Thorac Cardiovasc Surg 1998;10:117.

2

Vascular Disease

Abdominal Aortic Aneurysm

■ Essentials of Diagnosis

- Dilatation of the infrarenal aorta (>3 cm in diameter)
- Incidence increases with age and more common in men
- Most are asymptomatic until rupture; then 75% of patients die suddenly before reaching the hospital

■ Differential Diagnosis

- Tumor adjacent to aorta
- Pulsatile liver from tricuspid regurgitation
- Musculoskeletal back pain
- Acute abdomen (eg, pancreatitis)
- Aortic dissection
- Ureteric colic

■ Treatment

Less than 5.5 cm in diameter
- Watchful waiting
- Stop smoking
- Treat hypertension

Greater than 5.5 cm in diameter
- Repair unless risk is prohibitive
- Surgical replacement with a synthetic graft
- Endovascular repair with a percutaneous graft-stent combination is experimental but may be life-saving in nonsurgical candidates

■ Pearl

Abdominal aortic aneurysm shares some risk factors with atherosclerosis obliterans (male sex, smoking, age, hypertension) but is clearly not the same disease. Aortic aneurysm patients have different lipoprotein profiles and are less often diabetic. Also, genetic factors for aneurysm formation play a strong role.

Reference

The UK Small Aneurysm Trial Participants: Mortality results for randomized controlled trial of early elective surgery or ultrasonographic surveillance for small abdominal aortic aneurysms. Lancet 1998;352:1649.

Buerger Disease (Thromboangiitis Obliterans)

- **Essentials of Diagnosis**
    - An inflammatory vasculopathy (arteries and veins) that predominantly involves the hands and is invariably associated with smoking. Digital ulcers may be present.
    - Men older than 50 years
    - Thrombophlebitis may be the first sign of the disease
    - Angiography shows disease of the small and median arteries with corkscrew collaterals. Large arteries are unaffected.
    - Laboratory evidence of HLA antibodies (DR4, A9, B5, B8), increased complement activity, and anticollagen antibodies

- **Differential Diagnosis**
    - Atherosclerosis obliterans

- **Treatment**
    - Stop smoking
    - Prostaglandins may help ulcer healing

- **Pearl**

Buerger disease occasionally involves internal arteries, leading to internal organ problems such as acute myocardial infarction.

Reference

The European TAO Study Group: Oral iloprost in the treatment of thromboangiitis obliterans (Buerger's disease): A double blind, randomized, placebo controlled trial. Eur J Vasc Endovasc Surg 1998;15:300.

Cerebral Vascular Disease

- **Essentials of Diagnosis**
  - Rapid development of focal or global disturbance of cerebral function: duration less than 24 hours is a transient ischemic attack; greater than 24 hours is a stroke
  - Early computed tomography (CT) scan is negative, which excludes intracerebral or subarachnoid hemorrhage
  - Duplex ultrasound or angiography shows large-vessel disease

- **Differential Diagnosis**
  - Subdural hematoma
  - Epilepsy
  - Migraine
  - Hypoglycemia
  - Hypotension
  - Hypertensive encephalopathy
  - Cerebral infection
  - Brain tumor
  - Multiple sclerosis
  - Hysterical conversion

- **Treatment**
  - Transient ischemic attack: antiplatelet agents
  - Stroke: thrombolysis in appropriate candidates
  - Secondary prevention measures for atherosclerosis
  - Carotid surgery or stenting for symptomatic patients with greater than 70% diameter narrowing

- **Pearl**

Ischemic strokes in young patients without evidence of atherosclerosis may be due to focal carotid or cerebral artery dissection occurring spontaneously or from trauma.

Reference

MRC European Carotid Surgery Trial (ECST): Randomized trial of endarterectomy for recently symptomatic carotid stenosis: Final results of the MRC European Carotid Surgery Trial (ECST). Lancet 1998;351:1379.

Deep Venous Thrombosis

- **Essentials of Diagnosis**
  - Lower leg pain, swelling, erythema
  - Palpable chord, especially in the calf
  - Duplex ultrasound evidence of thrombus
  - Evidence of thrombus on CT or magnetic resonance angiography

- **Differential Diagnosis**
  - Ruptured Baker cyst
  - Abscesses
  - Ruptured plantaris tendon
  - Muscle strain
  - Tumors

- **Treatment**
  - Systemic anticoagulation for 3–6 months
  - Locally delivered thrombolysis in selected cases

- **Pearl**

Homan's sign (pain in the calf on dorsiflexion of the foot) is elicited by having the patient, not the examiner, dorsiflex the foot.

Reference

Levine M et al: A comparison of low molecular weight heparin administered primarily at home with unfractionated heparin administered in the hospital for proximal deep-vein thrombosis. N Engl J Med 1996;334:667.

Localized Lymphedema

- **Essentials of Diagnosis**
  - Isolated swollen extremity secondary to lymph vessel damage from surgery, radiation, disease, or trauma, or as a primary developmental abnormality
  - No evidence of heart failure, renal disease, malabsorption, or other edema-producing conditions

- **Differential Diagnosis**
  - Angioneurotic edema
  - Infectious lymphangitis
  - Venous insufficiency
  - Thrombophlebitis
  - Other causes of edema such as heart failure

- **Treatment**
  - Elevation of the limb and compressive stockings
  - Physiotherapy and massage
  - Meticulous skin care
  - Benzopyrone coumarin (not an anticoagulant)
  - Surgery in selected cases

- **Pearl**

Lymphedema precox represents 75% of cases of localized lymphedema, is more common in women, and usually begins at menarche or with the first pregnancy. Secondary localized lymphedema usually has its onset much later, when the diseases that cause it are more prevalent.

Reference

Mavile ME et al: Modified Charles operation for primary fibrosclerotic lymphedema. Lymphology 1994;27:14.

Peripheral Arterial Atherosclerosis Obliterans

- **Essentials of Diagnosis**
  - Intermittent claudication
  - Resting leg pain, ulceration, or gangrene
  - Reduced amplitude or absence of peripheral pulses
  - Ileofemoral bruits
  - Ankle-brachial artery pressure ratio less than 0.9
  - Cool feet when supine that blanch on elevation and become rubrous and warm when dependent

- **Differential Diagnosis**
  - Sciatica from lower back disease
  - Arterial embolism
  - Erythromelalgia
  - Vascular compartment compression syndromes

- **Treatment**
  - Stop smoking
  - Exercise
  - Angioplasty
  - Reconstructive surgery
  - Antiplatelet drugs—aspirin, clopidogrel, ticlopidine
  - Vasodilators—pentoxifylline, naftidrofuryl, prostacyclin analogues
  - Anticoagulants in selected cases
  - Vascular endothelial growth factor is experimental
  - Amputation

- **Pearl**

Loss of all hair on the dorsal aspect of the foot is a sign of markedly reduced blood flow.

Reference

Whyman MR, Ruckley CV: Should claudicants receive angioplasty or just exercise training? Surgery 1998;6:226.

Raynaud Phenomenon

- **Essentials of Diagnosis**
  - One or more digits blanch with cold exposure or emotional upset and subsequently show hyperemia when warmed
  - Nailfold capillaries are normal by microscopy in primary Raynaud phenomenon
  - Focal digital-tip necrosis

- **Differential Diagnosis**
  - Primary disease versus secondary causes such as collagen vascular diseases, vasoactive drugs, and blood viscosity disorders

- **Treatment**
  - Stop smoking
  - Avoid cold exposure
  - Avoid rings on affected digits
  - Use vasoactive drugs, such as calcium blockers and nitrates

- **Pearl**

Primary Raynaud phenomenon is 10 times more common in women; symptoms usually start at puberty and the thumb is rarely involved. Secondary Raynaud phenomenon begins at an older age, is less related to cold exposure, and more often involves the thumb.

Reference

Block JA, Sequeira W: Raynaud's phenomenon. Lancet 2001;357:2042.

Subclavian Coronary Artery Steal Syndrome

- ■ Essentials of Diagnosis
  - Status post coronary artery bypass grafting using an internal thoracic artery pedicle graft
  - Angina with unilateral arm exercise
  - Subclavian artery stenosis demonstrated by imaging, proximal to the internal thoracic artery used for the coronary graft, in the affected upper arm

- ■ Differential Diagnosis
  - Progressive native coronary artery disease
  - Technical problems with the internal thoracic artery graft
  - Disease in vein grafts to other coronary arteries

- ■ Treatment
  - Angioplasty and stenting of the subclavian artery
  - Extrathoracic surgical approach: conduit from carotid to the subclavian distal to the stenosis or distal subclavian to carotid anastomosis
  - Intrathoracic surgical approach: subclavian endarterectomy or aorto-subclavian grafting

- ■ Pearl

Because it is preferable to identify significant subclavian stenosis before doing internal thoracic artery pedicle grafts to the coronary arteries, a simple noninvasive technique can be used to identify patients for subclavian angiography: A systolic blood pressure difference between the arms greater than 15 mm Hg identifies most patients with significant unilateral subclavian disease.

Reference

Osborn LA et al: Screening for subclavian artery stenosis in patients who are candidates for coronary bypass surgery. Catheter Cardiovasc Interv 2002;56:162.

Superficial Thrombophlebitis

- **Essentials of Diagnosis**
  - Redness, swelling, and pain, usually in a preexisting varicose vein
  - Duplex ultrasound detection of thrombosis in a superficial vein

- **Differential Diagnosis**
  - Cellulitis
  - Insect bite
  - Trauma

- **Treatment**
  - Warm compresses
  - Nonsteroidal anti-inflammatory agents
  - Limb elevation

- **Pearl**

One quarter of patients with deep venous thrombosis have associated superficial thrombophlebitis; thus, an ultrasound exam should always be done for suspected superficial thrombophlebitis to exclude deep venous thrombosis, which requires systemic anticoagulation.

Reference

Chengelis DL et al: Progression of superficial thrombosis to deep venous thrombosis. J Vasc Surg 1996;24:745.

Superior Vena Cava Syndrome

- **Essentials of Diagnosis**
  - Facial swelling, headache, and arm edema
  - Prominent venous pattern may be seen over the anterior chest wall
  - Associated conditions may aid in the diagnosis, such as lung cancer, lymphoma, and indwelling catheter or pacemaker
  - Syndrome may be due to extrinsic compression (lung cancer) or de novo thrombosis (indwelling catheters)
  - Lung cancer used to be the most common cause. Causative factors are changing with increased utilization of indwelling catheters.
  - Venography is diagnostic. Magnetic resonance imaging, ultrasound, and CT may be alternates.

- **Differential Diagnosis & Causes**
  - Lung cancer
  - Lymphoma
  - Indwelling catheters and pacemaker leads
  - Fibrosing mediastinitis
  - Thoracic outlet syndrome
  - Retrosternal goiter

- **Treatment**
  - Depends on the cause:
    Malignancies; steroids, radiation, and chemotherapy
    Indwelling catheters and thrombosis; clot removal, angioplasty with stents
    Extrinsic compression: stents

- **Pearl**

Facial edema is an uncommon complaint. Superior vena cava syndrome must be excluded expeditiously when suspected.

Reference

Otten TR et al: Thromboembolic disease involving the superior vena cava and brachiocephalic veins. Chest 2003;123:809.

Takayasu Arteritis

- **Essentials of Diagnosis**
  - A severe inflammatory vascular disorder involving the aorta, its major branches, and the pulmonary artery
  - Predominantly found in Asian women less than 40 years old
  - Evidence of diffuse vascular disease (coronary, cerebral, peripheral), especially involving the upper extremities (pulseless disease)
  - Elevated erythrocyte sedimentation rate

- **Differential Diagnosis**
  - Diffuse atherosclerosis
  - Other vasculitides (eg, Buerger disease)

- **Treatment**
  - Corticosteroids
  - Percutaneous transluminal revascularization procedures
  - Vascular surgery

- **Pearl**

In East Indian patients, symptoms from involvement of the abdominal aorta and its branches are more common than in other patients.

Reference

Creager MA: Takayasu's arteritis. Rev Cardiovasc Med 2001;2:211.

Thoracic Aortic Aneurysm

- ■ Essentials of Diagnosis
  - • Ascending aortic diameter greater than 4 cm on imaging study
  - • Descending aortic diameter greater than 3.5 cm on imaging study

- ■ Differential Diagnosis
  - • Aortic dissection
  - • Aortic rupture with contained hematoma
  - • Mediastinal or thoracic tumor

- ■ Treatment
  - • Surgical replacement with a synthetic graft is considered in asymptomatic patients at the following diameters:

	Non-Marfan	Marfan
Ascending	5.5 cm	5.0 cm
Descending	6.5 cm	6.0 cm

  - • Endoluminal stent grafts are an alternative under investigation; long-term results are not yet known
  - • Symptomatic aneurysms (pain, impingement on other structures) need immediate replacement

- ■ Pearl

A careful family history with screening of blood relatives is important in aortic aneurysmal disease because one fifth of first-degree relatives of aneurysm patients have them also.

Reference

Davis RR et al: Yearly rupture/dissection rates for thoracic aortic aneurysms: Simple prediction based on size. Ann Thorac Surg 2002;73:291.

Thoracic Aortic Dissection

- **Essentials of Diagnosis**
  - Usually middle-aged or elderly hypertensive men; occasionally, young patients with history of Marfan syndrome or other connective tissue disorder; rarely, young women in late pregnancy or labor
  - Acute chest pain, frequently with hemodynamic instability
  - Possible shock, but usually normal or elevated blood pressure
  - Various neurologic symptoms, such as Horner syndrome, paraplegia, and stroke
  - Aortic regurgitation
  - Widened mediastinum on chest radiograph

- **Differential Diagnosis**
  - Acute myocardial infarction
  - Angina pectoris
  - Acute pericarditis
  - Pneumothorax
  - Pulmonary embolism
  - Boerhaave syndrome
  - Cerebrovascular accident
  - Acute surgical abdomen
  - Peripheral embolism
  - Neurologic disease causing paraplegia, Horner syndrome

- **Treatment**

  Acute management
  - Transfer to intensive care unit of tertiary care hospital without waiting for confirmatory imaging studies
  - Sodium nitroprusside intravenously (IV) to lower blood pressure acutely to the lowest level compatible with normal organ perfusion
  - Adjunctive IV beta-blockade to reduce aortic dP/dt

  Type B (distal dissection of descending thoracic aorta)
  - Uncomplicated: continued medical management
  - Complicated: endovascular stent graft placed percutaneously

  Type A (proximal dissection of ascending aorta)
  - Surgery to prevent aortic rupture, reestablish blood flow to occluded arteries, and correct aortic regurgitation if present

  Long-term management
  - Effective control of blood pressure and aortic dP/dt. Monitor aortic size and false lumen status periodically.

- **Pearl**

Patients with bicuspid aortic valve have a 9-fold higher risk of developing aortic dissection than those with normal aortic valves.

Reference

Sabik JF et al: Long-term effectiveness of operations for ascending aortic dissections. J Thorac Cardiovasc Surg 2000;119:946.

Venous Insufficiency

- **Essentials of Diagnosis**
  - Pain and swelling of the leg with prolonged standing
  - Dilated superficial veins (venous stars, varicose veins)
  - Increased skin pigmentation, lipodermatosclerosis
  - Ulcerations, usually on medial aspect of the lower leg
  - Duplex ultrasound to detect and locate refluxing segments

- **Differential Diagnosis**
  - Deep venous thrombosis
  - Phlegmasia cerulea dolens
  - Localized lymphedema
  - Enlarged inguinal lymph nodes obstructing flow
  - Heart failure

- **Treatment**
  - Apply compression stockings; elevate leg.
  - Isolated superficial vein insufficiency can be treated with sclerosis or vein stripping
  - Deep vein insufficiency can be treated surgically in selected patients

- **Pearl**

Isolated left-leg edema can be an early sign of congestive heart failure because venous pressures are normally higher in the left leg than the right, owing to mild compression of the left iliac vein by the right iliac artery crossing over it as it emerges from the aorta.

Reference

American Venous Forum Ad Hoc Committee: Classification and grading of chronic venous disease in the lower limbs. J Cardiovasc Surg 1997;38:437.

3

Valvular Heart Disease

Aortic Regurgitation, Acute

- ■ Essentials of Diagnosis
  - • Usually due to aortic dissection, endocarditis, or trauma
  - • Sudden severe dyspnea, orthopnea, and weakness
  - • Signs of pulmonary edema
  - • Soft first heart sound and short decrescendo aortic murmur
  - • Characteristic Doppler echocardiographic findings confirm aortic regurgitation (color jet), estimate its severity (short pressure half time), and estimate left ventricular pressure (premature closure of mitral valve, diastolic mitral regurgitation)

- ■ Differential Diagnosis
  - • Other causes of acute pulmonary edema
  - • Aorto-left ventricular fistula due to endocarditis

- ■ Treatment
  - • Prompt surgical intervention
  - • Sodium nitroprusside 0.3–10 µg/kg/min intravenously to support patient until surgery

- ■ Pearl

Acute aortic regurgitation does not cause the typical peripheral signs of chronic aortic regurgitation (eg, wide pulse pressure), and the diastolic murmur may be short and difficult to hear.

Reference

Ardehali A et al: Coronary blood flow reserve in acute aortic regurgitation. J Am Coll Cardiol 1995;25:1387.

Aortic Regurgitation, Chronic

- **Essentials of Diagnosis**
  - Following a long asymptomatic period, presentation with heart failure or angina
  - Wide pulse pressure with associated peripheral signs
  - Diastolic decrescendo murmur at the left sternal border
  - Left ventricular dilation and hypertrophy with preserved function
  - Presentation and findings depend on the rapidity of onset of regurgitation
  - Diagnosis confirmed and severity estimated by Doppler echocardiography or aortography

- **Differential Diagnosis**
  - Pulmonic regurgitation associated with high pulmonary pressures (Graham Steell murmur)
  - Patent ductus arteriosus
  - Mitral stenosis mimicking an Austin Flint murmur
  - Arteriovenous malformation with wide pulse pressure
  - Arteriovenous fistula near heart with continuous murmur
  - Left anterior descending coronary artery stenosis

- **Treatment**
  Mild to moderate aortic regurgitation
  - Give endocarditis prophylaxis
  - Control hypertension
  - Avoid heavy isometric exercise and competitive sports
  Moderate to severe aortic regurgitation
  - If symptomatic and left ventricular ejection fraction (LVEF) is greater than 25%, aortic valve replacement
  - If asymptomatic and LVEF is greater than 50%, oral vasodilator therapy
  - If asymptomatic and LVEF is 25–50%, aortic valve replacement

- **Pearl**

If the murmur of aortic regurgitation is loudest along the right sternal border, it suggests aortic root dilatation as the cause (Marfan syndrome, syphilis); the left sternal border suggests aortic leaflet diseases (rheumatic, ankylosing spondylitis).

Reference

Bonow RO: Chronic aortic regurgitation. Role of medical therapy and optimal timing for surgery. Cardiol Clin 1998;16:449.

Aortic Stenosis

- ■ Essentials of Diagnosis
  - • Angina pectoris
  - • Dyspnea (left ventricular heart failure)
  - • Effort syncope
  - • Systolic ejection murmur radiating to the carotid arteries
  - • Carotid upstroke delayed in reaching its peak and reduced in amplitude (parvus et tardus)
  - • Echocardiography shows thickened, immobile aortic valve leaflets
  - • Doppler echocardiography quantifies increased transvalvular pressure gradient and reduced valve area

- ■ Differential Diagnosis
  - • Discrete subvalvular aortic stenosis
  - • Supravalvular aortic stenosis
  - • Hypertrophic obstructive cardiomyopathy
  - • Pulmonic stenosis
  - • Ventricular septal defect

- ■ Treatment
  - • Endocarditis prophylaxis
  - • Dental hygiene
  - • Cholesterol-lowering therapy if appropriate
  - • Valve replacement surgery in symptomatic patients

- ■ Pearl

Vasodilators (eg, angiotensin-converting enzyme inhibitors, nitrates) and beta-blockers must be used with extreme caution if at all in patients with severe aortic stenosis, even if heart failure is present.

Reference

Aikawa K, Otto CM: Timing of surgery in aortic stenosis. Prog Cardiovasc Dis 2001;43:477.

Aortic Stenosis, Low Gradient, Low Output

- **Essentials of Diagnosis**
  - Severe aortic stenosis by valve area estimation (<1.0 cm^2)
  - Low transvalvular gradient (mean <40 mm Hg)
  - Depressed left ventricular systolic function (LVEF $<40\%$)
  - Transvalvular gradient, but not aortic valve area, increases with dobutamine infusion

- **Differential Diagnosis**
  - Mild to moderate aortic stenosis with left ventricular dysfunction (valve area increases with dobutamine)
  - Overestimation of stenosis severity because of failure to account for pressure recovery by Doppler echocardiography; cardiac catheterization will reveal the true valve area
  - Technical errors in calculating aortic valve area and measuring valve gradient by Doppler echocardiography (eg, failure to account for a subvalvular gradient and inaccurate left ventricular outflow tract measurement, resulting in underestimate)

- **Treatment**
  - Surgery if left ventricle responds to dobutamine and valve area remains severely reduced
  - Those with truly mild to moderate aortic stenosis should be treated for left ventricular dysfunction. Angiotensin-converting enzyme inhibitors are not contraindicated in this situation.

- **Pearl**

Overestimation of the severity of aortic valve stenosis by Doppler echocardiography because of unrecognized pressure recovery occurs most often when aortic stenosis is moderate and the ascending aorta is small (≤ 2 cm).

Reference

Connolly H et al: Severe aortic stenosis with low transvalvular gradient and severe left ventricular dysfunction. Results of aortic valve replacement in 52 patients. Circulation 2000;101:1940.

Aortic Stenosis, Subvalvular

- **Essentials of Diagnosis**
    - In the absence of other congenital heart abnormalities, it is usually asymptomatic
    - Low-pitched systolic ejection murmur is heard at the left sternal border radiating to the neck
    - Two-dimensional echocardiography defines the anatomy of the obstruction
    - Doppler echocardiography estimates the pressure gradient

- **Differential Diagnosis**
    - Valvular aortic stenosis
    - Supravalvular aortic stenosis
    - Hypertrophic cardiomyopathy

- **Treatment**
    - Endocarditis prophylaxis
    - Corrective surgery

- **Pearl**

Associated congenital heart defects are common, especially ventricular septal defect, patent ductus arteriosus, coarctation of the aorta, bicuspid aortic valve, and persistent left superior vena cava.

Reference

Bezold LI et al: Development and validation of an echocardiographic model for predicting progression of discrete subaortic stenosis in children. Am J Cardiol 1998;81:314.

Aortic Stenosis, Supravalvular

- **■ Essentials of Diagnosis**
  - Phenotypic and molecular evidence of Williams syndrome
  - Dyspnea on exertion and angina are common
  - Elevated blood pressure in the right arm versus left
  - Harsh systolic ejection murmur typical of valvular aortic stenosis
  - Associated aortic regurgitation, peripheral pulmonary artery stenosis, coarctation of the aorta, and mitral regurgitation are common
  - Doppler echocardiography defines the anatomy of the lesion and its severity

- **■ Differential Diagnosis**
  - Valvular aortic stenosis
  - Subvalvular aortic stenosis
  - Hypertrophic obstructive cardiomyopathy
  - Left subclavian artery stenosis
  - Coronary artery disease

- **■ Treatment**
  - Endocarditis prophylaxis
  - Surgical correction in symptomatic patients

- **■ Pearl**

Because the coronary arteries arise proximal to the obstruction, they display the same elevated pressure as the left ventricle, resulting in premature coronary atherosclerosis.

Reference

Eronen M et al: Cardiovascular manifestations in 75 patients with Williams syndrome. J Med Genet 2002;39:554.

Bicuspid Aortic Valve

- **Essentials of Diagnosis**
  - History of murmur since infancy, coarctation repair, or endocarditis
  - Early systolic ejection click, harsh crescendo-decrescendo systolic murmur, or early decrescendo diastolic murmur
  - Left ventricular hypertrophy
  - Abnormal bicuspid or dysplastic aortic valve with stenosis or regurgitation on Doppler echocardiography

- **Differential Diagnosis**
  - Discrete subaortic stenosis
  - Hypertrophic obstructive cardiomyopathy
  - Marfan syndrome with aortic regurgitation
  - Pulmonic stenosis
  - Ventricular septal defect
  - Mitral valve prolapse with mitral regurgitation

- **Treatment**
  - Antibiotic prophylaxis to prevent endocarditis
  - Dental hygiene
  - Avoidance of strenuous isometric exercise
  - Corrective surgery in symptomatic patients

- **Pearl**

The early systolic ejection sound differentiates bicuspid aortic valve from innocent systolic flow murmurs.

Reference

Ward C: Clinical significance of the bicuspid aortic valve. Heart 2000;83:81.

Infective Endocarditis

- **Essentials of Diagnosis**
  - Fever
  - Blood cultures positive for characteristic microbe or persistently positive blood cultures for compatible microbe
  - Characteristic cardiac lesions on echocardiography: oscillating mass, abscess, or prosthetic valve dehiscence

- **Differential Diagnosis**
  - Fever due to other causes
  - Sepsis not due to infective endocarditis
  - Valvular lesions on echocardiography that resemble vegetations (eg, myxomatous valves)

- **Treatment**
  - Appropriate antibiotic therapy
  - Cardiac surgery, usually to replace the infected valve(s) for: failure of antibiotic therapy, worsening valve dysfunction with heart failure, recurrent septic emboli, most prosthetic valve infections, intracardiac abscess or fistula, purulent pericarditis and endocarditis due to fungi or antibiotic-resistant gram-negative organisms

- **Pearl**

Septic pulmonary embolus means right-heart, usually tricuspid valve endocarditis, until proven otherwise. The murmur of tricuspid regurgitation with normal right-heart pressures is often unimpressive or absent.

Reference

Li JS et al: Proposed modifications to the Duke criterion for the diagnosis of infective endocarditis. Clin Infect Dis 2000;30:633.

Lutembacher Syndrome

- ■ Essentials of Diagnosis
  - • Congenital atrial septal defect plus rheumatic mitral stenosis

- ■ Differential Diagnosis
  - • Mitral stenosis with the opening snap mistaken for a wide fixed split second heart sound and another systolic murmur (eg, innocent flow, mild mitral or tricuspid regurgitation) mistaken for a pulmonary outflow murmur
  - • Atrial septal defect with the wide fixed split second heart sound mistaken for an opening snap and a tricuspid flow rumble mistaken for the murmur of mitral stenosis
  - • Ebstein anomaly of the tricuspid valve and an atrial septal defect

- ■ Treatment
  - • Mitral stenosis will increase the left to right shunt and further reduce left ventricular filling; expect an earlier onset of symptoms and need to repair
  - • It is possible to go through the atrial septal defect to perform catheter balloon valvuloplasty on the mitral valve and then place a percutaneous device to close the atrial septal defect, but experience is scant
  - • Corrective surgery is needed for both conditions

- ■ Pearl

A loud pulmonary outflow murmur and a fixed triple second heart sound (aortic, pulmonic, opening snap) suggest the presence of atrial septal defect with mitral stenosis.

Reference

Crawford MH: Iatrogenic Lutembacher's syndrome revisited. Circulation 1990;81:1422.

Mitral Regurgitation, Acute

- ■ Essentials of Diagnosis
  - • Sudden severe orthopnea
  - • Evidence of pulmonary edema
  - • Fourth heart sound
  - • Early systolic murmur due to rapid equilibration of left ventricular and left atrial pressures
  - • Doppler echocardiography establishes diagnosis, severity, and cause of mitral regurgitation

- ■ Differential Diagnosis
  - • Other causes of acute pulmonary edema not associated with mitral regurgitation
  - • Aortic stenosis with heart failure
  - • Mitral stenosis with heart failure

- ■ Treatment
  - • Stabilization with vasodilators, intra-aortic balloon pump
  - • Urgent surgical repair or replacement

- ■ Pearl

The most common cause of acute mitral regurgitation is chordal rupture, usually due to myxomatous changes in the valve structure. Patients with flail leaflets who are transiently in severe heart failure should be considered for surgical repair regardless of subsequent symptoms.

Reference

Ling LH et al: Clinical outcome of mitral regurgitation due to flail leaflet. N Engl J Med 1996;335:1417.

Mitral Regurgitation, Chronic Functional

- **Essentials of Diagnosis**
  - Major causes include ischemic heart disease and dilated cardiomyopathy
  - Dyspnea or orthopnea
  - Signs of left ventricular dysfunction
  - Characteristic apical systolic murmur
  - Doppler echocardiography shows dilated, dysfunctional left ventricle and a regurgitant jet into the left atrium

- **Differential Diagnosis**
  - Organic mitral regurgitation
  - Tricuspid regurgitation
  - Aortic stenosis
  - Ventricular septal defect

- **Treatment**
  - Endocarditis prophylaxis
  - Treatment of the underlying condition (eg, revascularization)
  - Treatment of left ventricular dysfunction, including vasodilator drugs
  - Oral anticoagulation
  - Surgical repair or replacement in selected cases

- **Pearl**

Although patients with concomitant ischemic heart disease and functional mitral regurgitation have a worse prognosis than patients with organic mitral regurgitation, mitral annuloplasty or other reparative techniques may improve outcomes after revascularization therapy and prevent future surgery in patients with moderate to severe mitral regurgitation due to ischemic heart disease.

Reference

Bolling SF et al: Intermediate-term outcome of mitral reconstruction in cardiomyopathy. J Thorac Cardiovasc Surg 1998;115:381.

Mitral Regurgitation, Chronic Organic

- **Essentials of Diagnosis**
  - Disease principally of the mitral valve leaflets caused by myxo-matous changes, rheumatic fever, collagen vascular disease, or endocarditis
  - Dyspnea or orthopnea
  - Characteristic apical systolic murmur
  - Doppler echocardiographic evidence of systolic regurgitation into the left atrium

- **Differential Diagnosis**
  - Functional mitral regurgitation
  - Aortic stenosis
  - Ventricular septal defect
  - Hypertrophic obstructive cardiomyopathy
  - Other causes of dyspnea and orthopnea

- **Treatment**
  - Rheumatic fever prophylaxis
  - Endocarditis prophylaxis
  - Treatment for heart failure
  - Oral anticoagulation for atrial fibrillation
  - Surgical repair or replacement in symptomatic patients or those with severe regurgitation and left ventricular dysfunction

- **Pearl**

Afterload, or the left ventricular wall tension after the aortic valve has opened, is not increased in chronic mitral regurgitation because of the low impedance leak into the left atrium. Consequently, lowering it further with vasodilators will only reduce forward blood flow, worsening the patient's overall hemodynamic status.

Reference

Tribouilloy CM et al: Impact of preoperative symptoms on survival after surgical correction of organic mitral regurgitation: Rationale for optimizing surgical indications. Circulation 1999;99:400.

Mitral Stenosis

- **Essentials of Diagnosis**

    - Exertional dyspnea, paroxysmal nocturnal dyspnea, orthopnea, or fatigue (later stages)
    - Opening snap, loud first heart sound (closing snap), diastolic rumbling murmur; with pulmonary hypertension, a parasternal lift with a loud pulmonic component of the second heart sound
    - Electrocardiographic evidence of left atrial enlargement or atrial fibrillation; right ventricular hypertrophy in later stages
    - Radiographic signs of left atrial enlargement and normal left ventricular size
    - Thickened mitral valve leaflets with restricted valve motion and reduced orifice area demonstrated on 2-dimensional echocardiography
    - Elevated transmitral pressure gradient and prolonged pressure half-time by Doppler echocardiography

- **Differential Diagnosis**

    - Tricuspid stenosis
    - Aortic regurgitation with prominent Austin Flint murmur
    - Other causes of left-heart failure
    - Other causes of pulmonary hypertension
    - Left atrial myxoma, thrombus, vegetation
    - Cor triatriatum

- **Treatment**

    All patients
    - Rheumatic fever prophylaxis
    - Endocarditis prophylaxis
    - Diuretics for heart failure; vasodilators relatively contraindicated
    - Warfarin for history of systemic emboli or atrial fibrillation
    - Digitalis, beta-blockers, or calcium channel blockers for rate control in atrial fibrillation
    Symptomatic patients with moderate to severe mitral stenosis
    - Percutaneous mitral balloon valvoplasty
    - Surgical commissurotomy (open or closed)
    - Mitral valve replacement

- **Pearl**

Severe mitral stenosis can present as hemoptysis because of elevated pressures in the bronchial veins from the effects of pulmonary hypertension on systemic venous pressure.

Reference

Iung B et al: Late results of percutaneous mitral commissurotomy in a series of 1024 patients. Analysis of late clinical deterioration: Frequency, anatomic findings, and predictive factors. Circulation 1999;99:3272.

Mitral Valve Prolapse

■ Essentials of Diagnosis

- Organic mitral regurgitation due to myxomatous changes in the valve leaflets and chordae
- Most patients are asymptomatic
- Characteristic midsystolic click and late systolic apical murmur that change in intensity and timing with bedside maneuvers that alter left ventricular volume
- Doppler echocardiography shows systolic prolapse of the redundant mitral leaflets into the left atrium with late systolic mitral regurgitation

■ Differential Diagnosis

- Aortic stenosis
- Ventricular septal defect
- Hypertrophic obstructive cardiomyopathy
- Functional mitral regurgitation

■ Treatment

- Endocarditis prophylaxis
- Surgical repair or replacement for moderate to severe regurgitation if symptoms are present or left ventricular function is impaired

■ Pearl

The best bedside maneuver for identifying the murmur of mitral valve prolapse is the stand-squat with cardiac auscultation. Standing decreases left ventricular volume, causing the click-murmur complex to occur earlier in systole, and squatting produces the opposite effects.

Reference

Freed LA et al: Prevalence and clinical outcome of mitral-valve prolapse. N Engl J Med 1999;341:1.

Mixed Aortic & Mitral Valve Disease

- ■ Essentials of Diagnosis
  - • Moderate aortic regurgitation and mitral regurgitation
  - • Moderate aortic stenosis and mitral stenosis
  - • Moderate aortic stenosis and mitral regurgitation
  - • Moderate aortic regurgitation and mitral stenosis

- ■ Differential Diagnosis
  - • Mild valve disease
  - • Severe valve disease will dominate management
  - • The murmur of moderate to severe tricuspid regurgitation may be mimicked by moderate aortic stenosis or mitral regurgitation

- ■ Treatment
  - • Aortic regurgitation/mitral regurgitation: The combined volume load on the left ventricle will accelerate the development of left ventricular failure; use mitral regurgitation guidelines for surgery in asymptomatic patients. The role of vasodilators is uncertain.
  - • Aortic stenosis/mitral stenosis: Mitral stenosis restricts left ventricular filling and impairs the ability to compensate for aortic stenosis by increasing pressure. Expect earlier onset of symptoms for any given severity of aortic stenosis.
  - • Aortic stenosis/mitral regurgitation: Mitral regurgitation compromises ability to increase left ventricular systolic pressure and maintain forward stroke volume, and aortic stenosis increases filling pressures leading to pulmonary congestion. Expect earlier onset of symptoms than with either lesion alone.
  - • Aortic regurgitation/mitral stenosis: Left ventricular filling is maintained by aortic regurgitation but less than expected for the degree of aortic regurgitation because of mitral stenosis. Mitral stenosis usually dominates the picture and dictates surgery for pulmonary congestion. Vasodilator drugs are probably of little value.

- ■ Pearl

Moderate to severe aortic regurgitation can result in a diastolic rumble at the apex called the Austin Flint murmur; don't mistake it for mitral stenosis.

Reference

Choudhary SK et al: Fate of mild aortic valve disease after mitral valve intervention. J Thorac Cardiovasc Surg 2001;122:583.

Mixed Aortic Valve Disease

- **Essentials of Diagnosis**
  - Moderate aortic regurgitation and estimated aortic valve area 0.8 to 1.2 cm^2 (moderate aortic stenosis)

- **Differential Diagnosis**
  - Mild aortic regurgitation or mild aortic stenosis
  - Severe aortic regurgitation or aortic stenosis; the severe lesion dominates management
  - The murmur of patent ductus arteriosus may be mimicked by moderate aortic stenosis/aortic regurgitation

- **Treatment**
  - The combined pressure/volume load on the left ventricle will accelerate left ventricular failure; consider surgery in asymptomatic patients with an ejection fraction of 50–60% or left ventricular end-diastolic volume greater than 150 mL/m^2
  - Vasodilator drugs are contraindicated because of aortic stenosis

- **Pearl**

Moderate to severe aortic regurgitation is almost always accompanied by a loud systolic ejection murmur due to increased stroke volume. Don't mistake this for aortic stenosis at the bedside; pay attention to the carotid pulse and the peripheral signs of aortic regurgitation.

Reference

Attenhofer Jost CH et al: Echocardiography in the evaluation of systolic murmurs of unknown cause. Am J Med 2000;108:614.

Mixed Mitral Valve Disease

- ■ Essentials of Diagnosis
  - • Rheumatic mitral valve disease with moderate mitral regurgitation and a mean mitral diastolic gradient greater than 10 mm Hg and valve area of 1.1 to 1.5 cm^2 (moderate mitral stenosis)

- ■ Differential Diagnosis
  - • Mild mitral regurgitation or mild mitral stenosis
  - • Severe mitral regurgitation or mitral stenosis; the severe lesion dominates management

- ■ Treatment
  - • Mitral valvuloplasty is contraindicated
  - • Treat per mitral regurgitation guidelines
  - • The combined pressure/volume load on the left atrium increases the likelihood of atrial fibrillation, which is an indication for surgery

- ■ Pearl

Moderate to severe mitral regurgitation may be associated with a short mid-diastolic rumble due to the large diastolic flow volume returning from the left atrium. Don't mistake this for mitral stenosis; pay attention to an opening snap or signs of a longer, harsher diastolic rumble.

Reference

Mavioglu I et al: Valve repair for rheumatic mitral disease. J Heart Valve Dis 2001;10:596.

Periprosthetic Valve Leaks

- **Essentials of Diagnosis**
  - New murmur in a patient with a prosthetic valve or a regurgitant murmur ascribed to the prosthetic valve
  - Echocardiographic evidence of perivalvular leak
  - Clinical deterioration, embolism, or hemolysis

- **Differential Diagnosis**
  - Prosthetic valve malfunction: thrombus, vegetation, or pannus
  - Infective endocarditis
  - Hemolysis due to prosthesis malfunction or other causes
  - Embolism from thrombus formation
  - Clinical deterioration for other reasons (eg, prosthesis too small)

- **Treatment**
  - Severe periprosthetic leak may require redo operation
  - Infective endocarditis almost always necessitates surgery
  - Transcatheter occlusion devices are being perfected
  - Medical therapy is effective in less than severe cases; beta-blockers are recommended to reduce shear forces

- **Pearl**

Marked anemia due to perivalvular leak–induced hemolysis must be corrected immediately by transfusion. This will increase the viscosity of the blood, reduce turbulent flow through the leak, and decrease hemolysis. In some patients, this may be sufficient to stop hemolysis and avoid a reparative procedure.

Reference

Garcia MJ et al: Mechanisms of hemolysis with mitral prosthetic regurgitation. J Am Coll Cardiol 1996;27:399.

Pulmonic Regurgitation

- ■ Essentials of Diagnosis
  - • Diastolic murmur at the left upper sternal border that increases with inspiration
  - • Loud pulmonic component of second heart sound
  - • Characteristic Doppler echocardiographic findings

- ■ Differential Diagnosis
  - • Aortic regurgitation
  - • Tricuspid stenosis
  - • Right-heart failure from other causes

- ■ Treatment
  - • Eradication of underlying cause such as pulmonary hypertension or infective endocarditis
  - • Pulmonic valve replacement

- ■ Pearl

Trivial to mild pulmonic regurgitation is present by color Doppler echocardiography in almost all adults and is of no clinical consequence.

Reference

Shively BK: Transesophageal echocardiographic (TEE) evaluation of the aortic valve, left ventricular outflow tract, and pulmonic valve. Cardiol Clin 2000;18:711.

Pulmonic Stenosis

- **Essentials of Diagnosis**
  - Systolic murmur at the left second intercostal space preceded by a systolic click
  - Reduced intensity of pulmonic component of second heart sound
  - Characteristic echocardiographic findings

- **Differential Diagnosis**
  - Aortic stenosis
  - Ventricular septal defect
  - Right-heart failure from other causes

- **Treatment**
  - Antibiotic prophylaxis for infective endocarditis
  - Balloon valvuloplasty
  - Pulmonary valve replacement

- **Pearl**

The ejection sound associated with pulmonic valve stenosis is the only right-sided auscultatory sign that decreases in intensity with inspiration.

Reference

Rao PS et al: Results of 3 to 10 year follow up of balloon dilation of the pulmonic valve. Heart 1998;80:591.

Rheumatic Fever, Acute

- **Essentials of Diagnosis**
  - Carditis in almost half: heart failure, new organic heart murmur (mitral regurgitation), pericarditis
  - Evidence of streptococcal infection: throat culture, detection of streptococcal antibodies
  - Chorea
  - Migratory arthritis
  - Typical skin findings: subcutaneous nodules, erythema marginatum

- **Differential Diagnosis**
  - Juvenile rheumatic arthritis
  - Infective endocarditis
  - Myocarditis due to other causes
  - Pericarditis due to other causes
  - Mitral valve prolapse

- **Treatment**
  - Penicillin, sulfadiazine, erythromycin, or azithromycin
  - Aspirin for arthritis
  - Corticosteroids relieve symptoms, but no evidence of reduced residual damage
  - Antibiotic prophylaxis for streptococcal infections until risk is minimal (ie, age >40 years without exposure to children)

- **Pearl**

Although the peak incidence of acute rheumatic fever is at age 12 years, it can occur at any age and recurrences are common, especially during pregnancy.

Reference

Ferrieri P et al: Proceedings of the Jones Criteria workshop. Circulation 2002;106:2521.

Tricuspid Regurgitation

- ■ Essentials of Diagnosis
  - • Prominent *v* wave in jugular venous pulse
  - • Systolic murmur at left lower sternal border that increases with inspiration
  - • Characteristic Doppler echocardiographic findings

- ■ Differential Diagnosis
  - • Mitral regurgitation
  - • Other causes of elevated neck veins

- ■ Treatment
  - • Reduction in pulmonary artery pressure
  - • Sodium restriction and diuretics for venous congestion
  - • Surgical repair or replacement for severe regurgitation in symptomatic patients

- ■ Pearl

The murmur of tricuspid regurgitation varies with the level of right ventricular pressure. Low-pressure tricuspid regurgitation causes a short early systolic murmur that is often confused with an innocent flow murmur. When pressures are high, the murmur mimics that of mitral regurgitation.

Reference

Shatapathy P et al: Tricuspid valve repair: A rational alternative. J Heart Valve Dis 2000;9:276.

Tricuspid Stenosis

■ **Essentials of Diagnosis**
- Almost always accompanies rheumatic mitral stenosis, but can be due to carcinoid heart disease
- Prominent *a* wave and reduced *y* descent in jugular venous pulse
- Diastolic murmur at left lower sternal border that increases with inspiration
- Characteristic Doppler echocardiographic findings

■ **Differential Diagnosis**
- Mitral stenosis
- Right arterial myxoma
- Metastatic tumors to right heart
- Pulmonary hypertension with right-heart failure

■ **Treatment**

All patients
- Endocarditis prophylaxis
- Rheumatic fever prophylaxis

Symptomatic patients
- Percutaneous balloon valvotomy
- Surgical intervention, usually in combination with mitral valve surgery

■ **Pearl**

Surgical intervention can be successful in patients with carcinoid syndrome because this tumor may have a prolonged course and respond to medical therapy.

Reference

Sancaktar O et al: Late results of combined percutaneous balloon valvuloplasty of mitral and tricuspid valves. Cathet Cardiovasc Diagn 1998;45:246.

4

Cardiomyopathy/Heart Failure

Alcoholic Cardiomyopathy

- ■ Essentials of Diagnosis
  - Heavy and continuous alcohol consumption: 80 g/d for 10 years
  - Symptoms and signs of biventricular congestive heart failure
  - Proximal myopathy is common
  - Regression of cardiomegaly with alcohol cessation

- ■ Differential Diagnosis
  - Certain heavy metals (cobalt, lead, iron) found in illegally produced alcoholic beverages
  - Metabolic disturbances in alcoholics: hypermagnesemia, hypokalemia, selenium deficiency, thiamine deficiency
  - Hypertensive heart disease; common in alcoholics
  - Other causes of cardiomyopathy

- ■ Treatment
  - Cessation of alcohol consumption
  - Correction of metabolic and nutritional deficiencies
  - Treatment of hypertension
  - General therapy of heart failure
  - Transplantation is feasible in abstinent individuals

- ■ Pearl

An early clue to the presence of alcoholic cardiomyopathy is the development of left ventricular hypertrophy on electrocardiogram (ECG) with normal systolic function by echocardiography.

Reference

Nicolas JM et al: The effect of controlled drinking in alcoholic cardiomyopathy. Ann Intern Med 2002;16:192.

Cardiac Cachexia

- **Essentials of Diagnosis**
  - Chronic severe heart failure
  - Unintentional loss of more than 6% of previous nonedematous weight with body mass index less than 24 kg/m^2
  - Muscle wasting, weakness
  - Decreased serum transferrin and elevated triglycerides

- **Differential Diagnosis**
  - Cancer
  - Hyperthyroidism
  - Acquired immunodeficiency syndrome
  - Intentional weight loss
  - Diuresis
  - Starvation

- **Treatment**
  - Nutritional support
  - Exclude digoxin toxicity
  - Exercise training

- **Pearl**

Overreliance on the patient's weight to manage heart failure can lead to serious errors. Fluid accumulation may be balanced by loss of lean body mass, masking worsening heart failure and the development of cardiac cachexia.

Reference

Anker SD et al: Prognostic importance of weight loss in chronic heart failure and the effect of angiotensin-converting enzyme inhibitors: An observational study. Lancet 2003;361:1077.

Cardiogenic Shock

- **Essentials of Diagnosis**
  - Tissue hypoperfusion, depressed mental status, cool extremities, urine output less than 30 mL/h
  - Hypotension: systolic blood pressure less than 80 mm Hg
  - Cardiac index less than 2.2 L/min/m^2
  - Pulmonary artery wedge pressure more than 18 mm Hg

- **Differential Diagnosis**
  - Septic shock
  - Hypovolemia
  - Cardiac tamponade

- **Treatment**

  Intubation, ventilation, and oxygen supplementation
  Swan-Ganz catheter
  - Pulmonary wedge pressure less than 18 mm Hg: administer fluids
  - Pulmonary wedge pressure greater than 18 mm Hg: administer inotropic agents

  ECG, echocardiogram
  - Acute myocardial infarction: coronary intervention if feasible
  - No myocardial infarction: hemodynamic management

  Inotropic agents
  - Dobutamine: 2–20 µg/kg/min intravenously (IV) or
  - Milrinone: load with 50 µg/kg IV over 10 minutes, then 0.375–0.75 µg/kg/min

  Intra-aortic balloon pump to stabilize for coronary intervention

- **Pearl**

  Successful myocardial revascularization is the only therapy that has been shown in prospective randomized trials to reduce mortality.

Reference

Hasdai D et al: Cardiogenic shock complicating acute coronary syndromes. Lancet 2000;356:749.

Cardiomyopathy, Idiopathic Dilated

- **Essentials of Diagnosis**
  - Systolic dysfunction with ventricular enlargement; symptoms of heart failure develop later in the disease
  - No evidence of ischemic heart disease, valvular heart disease, sustained hypertension, alcoholism, or other causative factor is found for cardiomyopathy
  - Estimated prevalence rate is 0.04%
  - Disease is 3 times more common in blacks and males as in whites and females
  - Familial linkage is frequent and may be close to 20%

- **Differential Diagnosis**
  - Ischemic cardiomyopathy
  - Valvular heart disease
  - Hypertensive heart disease
  - Alcoholic cardiomyopathy
  - Cardiomyopathy related to thyroid dysfunction
  - Human immunodeficiency virus (HIV) cardiomyopathy

- **Treatment**
  - Angiotensin-converting enzyme inhibitors and beta-blockers
  - Diuretics and digoxin for symptomatic relief
  - Spironolactone for advanced heart failure
  - Cardiac resynchronization therapy in patients meeting criteria
  - Implantable cardioverter-defibrillator in survivors of sudden death and patients with unexplained syncope
  - Cardiac transplantation in patients with progressive disease despite optimal therapy (if transplantation criteria are met)

- **Pearl**

Prognosis is much better than with ischemic cardiomyopathy. Also, beta-blocker therapy will normalize left ventricular function in 10% of patients.

Reference

Cooper LT Jr, Gersh BJ: Viral infection, inflammation, and the risk of idiopathic dilated cardiomyopathy: Can the fire be extinguished? Am J Cardiol 2002;90:751.

Cardiomyopathy, Peripartum

- **Essentials of Diagnosis**
  - Development of heart failure during pregnancy or within 6 months of delivery
  - No identifiable cause
  - Reduced left ventricular systolic function

- **Differential Diagnosis**
  - Heart failure due to other causes
  - Pulmonary embolus
  - Aortic dissection with coronary artery compromise or cardiac tamponade

- **Treatment**
  - Angiotensin-converting enzyme inhibitors are contraindicated prepartum, but should be used postpartum
  - Prepartum hydralazine, nitrates, and digoxin are valuable
  - Anticoagulants are indicated because of the high risk of thromboemboli and should be continued until left ventricular function improves
  - Because peripartum cardiomyopathy is often reversible, left ventricular assist devices should be considered for severe cases
  - Cardiac transplantation may be needed
  - Avoid subsequent pregnancies

- **Pearl**

Because most cases occur within 1 month before or after delivery, early prepartum heart failure should raise suspicion of another cause, such as cocaine use. Special considerations for delivering a healthy baby in cocaine-addicted mothers are important.

Reference

Ostrzega E, Elkoyam U: Risk of subsequent pregnancy in women with a history of peripartum cardiomyopathy: Results of a survey. Circulation 1995;92 (suppl 1):1.

Cardiomyopathy, Restrictive

- **Essentials of Diagnosis**
  - Symptoms and signs of heart failure with predominantly right-sided findings
  - Normal left and right ventricular size and systolic function with dilated atria
  - Abnormalities of diastolic ventricular function suggestive of reduced ventricular compliance
  - Increased ventricular filling pressure (left > right) and reduced cardiac output
  - Evidence of a systemic disease that can infiltrate the heart (eg, amyloidosis, hemochromatosis, sarcoidosis, or glycogen storage disease)

- **Differential Diagnosis**
  - Dilated cardiomyopathy with restrictive physiology
  - Hypertrophic cardiomyopathy
  - Constrictive pericarditis

- **Treatment**
  - Diuresis to prevent pulmonary and systolic congestion
  - Maintenance of sinus rhythm to preserve atrial contribution to left ventricular filling
  - Rate control, if atrial fibrillation persists, to provide adequate time for left ventricular filling
  - Pacing for extreme bradycardia or conduction block
  - Management of ventricular tachyarrhythmias
  - Anticoagulation for those with atrial fibrillation and endocardial fibrosis
  - Treatment of the underlying systemic disease
  - Cardiac transplantation
  - Surgical resection of endocardial fibrosis in selected cases

- **Pearl**

Thick myocardial walls on ECG with normal or low-voltage ECG QRS complexes suggests infiltrative cardiomyopathy.

Reference

Kushwaha SS et al: Restrictive cardiomyopathy. N Engl J Med 1997;336:267.

Cardiomyopathy, Tachycardia Induced

- **Essentials of Diagnosis**
  - Typical dilated cardiomyopathy with reduced systolic function and
  - Ventricular or supraventricular tachycardia (not sinus tachycardia) for more than 15% of the day

- **Differential Diagnosis**
  - Idiopathic dilated cardiomyopathy should be suspected if left ventricular function does not improve with control or termination of the tachyarrhythmia
  - Other forms of heart failure with sinus tachycardia

- **Treatment**
  - Pharmacologic therapy or atrioventricular node ablation plus a pacemaker to control the rate
  - Cardioversion of ventricular tachycardia, atrial fibrillation, or atrial flutter
  - Pharmacologic therapy or ablation to eliminate the tachycardia

- **Pearl**

Tachyarrhythmias may contribute to decompensation in patients with underlying cardiac disease.

Reference

Aguinaga L et al: Long-term follow-up in patients with the permanent form of junctional reciprocating tachycardia treated with radiofrequency ablation. Pacing Clin Electrophysiol 1998;21:2073.

Cardiomyopathy, Tako-Tsubo

- ■ Essentials of Diagnosis
  - Transient left ventricular apical ballooning, possibly secondary to neurogenic stunned myocardium induced by emotional or physical stress
  - Changes in ST-T segment in several leads in ECG
  - No history of myocardial infarction, valvular heart disease, subarachnoid hemorrhage, or pheochromocytoma
  - No significant stenosis or slow flow in epicardial coronary arteries on angiography
  - Normal coronary flow reserve
  - Technetium-99m tetrofosmin tomographic imaging may reveal decreased uptake at the apex of the left ventricle

- ■ Differential Diagnosis
  - Acute myocardial infarction
  - Myocarditis
  - Cardiomyopathy following subarachnoid hemorrhage

- ■ Treatment
  - Spontaneous recovery in 2 weeks

- ■ Pearl

Not all ST elevations are secondary to myocardial injury. Pericarditis and early repolarization are in the differential diagnosis. Tako-tsubo cardiomyopathy is a rare cause of ST-T wave change in the western world.

Reference

Kurisu S et al: Tako-tsubo-like left ventricular dysfunction with ST-segment elevation: A novel cardiac syndrome mimicking acute myocardial infarction. Am Heart J 2002;143:448.

Chagas Heart Disease

- ■ Essentials of Diagnosis
  - • Remote history of residence in rural Central or South America
  - • ECG evidence of conduction system disease, especially right bundle branch block and left anterior fascicular block, and ST-segment elevation suggesting ventricular aneurysm
  - • Premature ventricular contractions and nonsustained ventricular tachycardia
  - • Echocardiographic evidence of an apical left ventricular aneurysm
  - • Positive serology for Chagas disease

- ■ Differential Diagnosis
  - • Coronary artery disease
  - • Dilated cardiomyopathy
  - • Isolated conduction system disease
  - • Other causes of ventricular arrhythmias

- ■ Treatment
  - • Heart failure: standard therapy is helpful
  - • Ventricular arrhythmias: amiodarone is very effective; implanted cardioverter-defibrillator, catheterization, or aneurysmectomy in selected cases
  - • Conduction disease: a pacemaker is often required
  - • Heart transplantation is feasible

- ■ Pearl

Left bundle branch block is more common in idiopathic dilated cardiomyopathy or coronary artery disease than in Chagas disease. Right bundle branch block with left anterior fascicular block suggests Chagas disease in patients with positive epidemiology and no evidence of coronary artery disease.

Reference

Davila DF et al: Effects of metoprolol in chagasic patients with severe congestive heart failure. Int J Cardiol 2002;85:255.

Chemotherapy-Induced Cardiac Disease

- ■ **Essentials of Diagnosis**
  - Anthracycline antibiotics (doxorubicin, daunorubicin) are the most common agents associated with cardiotoxicity; chronic cardiomyopathy is common with increasing cumulative dosage (>400 mg/m^2); acute myopericarditis is rare; QT_c prolongation is the most common acute effect
  - 5-Fluorouracil may cause vaso-occlusive complications, particularly acute myocardial infarction. Cisplatin, bleomycin, and vinca alkaloids may also cause myocardial infarction secondary to vasospastic effects.
  - Cyclophosphamide (>2000 mg/m^2) may cause severe cardiomyopathy; interferon-alpha and trastuzumab rarely cause cardiomyopathy
  - Interleukin-2 may cause capillary leak syndrome, noncardiogenic pulmonary edema, and occasionally myocardial infarction

- ■ **Differential Diagnosis & Monitoring**
  - Radionuclide ventriculography or echocardiography detects decreased ejection fraction, but significant myocardium may be irretrievably lost by the time of reduced ejection fraction
  - Echocardiographic rate of relaxation and fractional shortening of diastolic filling may detect early-onset cardiomyopathy
  - Dobutamine echocardiography and exercise radionuclide angiography may predict late-onset cardiac dysfunction in patients with normal resting cardiac function
  - Coexistent cardiomyopathy such as ischemic and dilated cardiomyopathies should be in the differential diagnosis

- ■ **Prevention & Treatment**
  - Limit the dose of anthracycline and use new formulations (liposome-encapsulated)
  - Calcium channel blockers, beta-blockers, and iron-chelating agents are cardioprotective
  - Modified dosing schedules may also be protective
  - Other agents may be cardioprotective, such as probucol, mesna, and vitamin E
  - Once cardiomyopathy develops, prognosis is poor and treatment is similar to that for heart failure

- ■ **Pearl**

Patients receiving cardiotoxic chemotherapy must undergo periodic noninvasive cardiac assessment, and early indicators should lead to discontinuation of cardiotoxic chemotherapy.

Reference

Gharib MI, Burnett AK: Chemotherapy-induced cardiotoxicity: Current practice and prospects of prophylaxis. Eur J Heart Fail 2002;4:235.

Congestive Heart Failure Due Predominantly to Diastolic Dysfunction

- **Essentials of Diagnosis**
  - Clinical presentation of congestive heart failure
  - Normal left ventricular systolic function
  - Abnormal left ventricular diastolic function

- **Differential Diagnosis**
  - Pulmonary hypertension
  - Mitral valve disease
  - Transient myocardial ischemia
  - Volume overload

- **Treatment**
  - Diuretics
  - Beta-blockers
  - Dihydropyridine calcium channel blockers
  - Treatment of underlying cause (eg, hypertension, myocardial ischemia)
  - Antiarrhythmia drugs to preserve sinus rhythm

- **Pearl**

Heart failure due to diastolic dysfunction is often a diagnosis of exclusion when echocardiography shows normal systolic function. If echocardiography does not reveal marked diastolic dysfunction, suspect acute transient myocardial ischemia as the cause of heart failure.

Reference

Argeja B, Grossman W: Evaluation and management of diastolic heart failure. Circulation 2003;107:659.

Congestive Heart Failure Due Predominantly to Systolic Left Ventricular Dysfunction

■ **Essentials of Diagnosis**

- Dyspnea on exertion, paroxysmal nocturnal dyspnea, orthopnea and dyspnea at rest (late stage)
- Jugular vein distention, peripheral edema, sinus tachycardia, pulmonary rales, cardiomegaly, third heart sound, and liver enlargement
- Left ventricular systolic dysfunction

■ **Differential Diagnosis**

- Chronic lung disease
- Pneumonia
- Pulmonary emboli
- Pericardial disease—tamponade or constriction
- Nephrosis
- Hepatic cirrhosis
- Hypothyroidism

■ **Treatment**

- Diuretics
- Digoxin
- Angiotensin-converting enzyme inhibitors
- Angiotensin-receptor blockers
- Beta-blockers
- Direct vasodilators
- Aldosterone antagonists
- Antiarrhythmic drugs
- Automatic implantable cardioverter-defibrillator
- Biventricular pacing
- Revascularization or other anti-ischemic therapy
- Ventricular aneurysmectomy
- Exercise training
- Cardiac transplantation
- Anticoagulation

■ **Pearl**

Elevated systemic venous pressure due to heart failure may produce pleural effusions, which can accumulate preferentially in the major and minor fissures of the lungs, leading to an appearance of a pulmonary mass or "pseudo-tumor" that disappears with diuresis.

Reference

Drazner MH et al: Prognostic importance of elevated jugular venous pressure and a third heart sound in patients with heart failure. N Engl J Med 2001;345:574.

Cor Pulmonale/Right-Heart Failure

- **Essentials of Diagnosis**
  - Right ventricular dysfunction (on echocardiography) due to lung disease
  - Acute right-heart failure accompanying acute respiratory failure, usually due to chronic obstructive lung disease
  - Chronic right-heart failure due to pulmonary hypertension
  - Hypoxia almost always present when breathing room air
  - Normal or near normal left ventricular function and filling pressures

- **Differential Diagnosis**
  - Right-heart failure due to left-heart failure
  - Right ventricular myocardial infarction
  - Constrictive pericarditis
  - Other cardiac causes of right-heart failure, such as pulmonic stenosis or atrial septal defect

- **Treatment**
  - Oxygen
  - Diuretics
  - Correction of bronchospasm or other reversible pulmonary conditions
  - Angiotension-converting enzyme inhibitors have not been beneficial. Beta-blockers and digoxin must be used with caution.

- **Pearl**

ECG evidence of right ventricular enlargement or hypertrophy despite optimal treatment of the patient's pulmonary condition suggests a very poor prognosis and should be taken into consideration in treatment planning.

Reference

Incalzi RA et al: Electrocardiographic signs of chronic cor pulmonale: A negative prognostic finding in chronic obstructive pulmonary disease. Circulation 1999;99:1600.

Hemochromatosis & the Heart

- **Essentials of Diagnosis**
  - Autosomal recessive iron-storage disease involves the heart as well as the pancreas, skin, liver, and gonads
  - Disease is primary, or secondary to multiple transfusions
  - Disease usually causes dilated cardiomyopathy, but may cause restrictive cardiomyopathy
  - Conduction abnormalities and supraventricular and ventricular arrhythmias occur in one third of patients
  - Fasting transferrin saturation greater than 50–60% is a sensitive screening test

- **Differential Diagnosis**
  - Idiopathic dilated cardiomyopathy
  - Idiopathic restrictive cardiomyopathy

- **Treatment**
  - Phlebotomy (cardiomyopathy may show dramatic recovery)
  - Iron chelation with desferrioxamine
  - Cardiac transplantation in advanced cases

- **Pearl**

This is a potentially reversible cardiomyopathy. Early recognition is crucial for successful treatment.

Reference

Little DR: Hemochromatosis: Diagnosis and management. Am Fam Physician 1996;53:2623.

High-Altitude Pulmonary Edema

■ Essentials of Diagnosis
  - Rapid ascent to altitude over 7200 feet
  - Symptoms and signs of pulmonary edema
  - Likelihood increased by higher elevations, vigorous physical activity, alcohol consumption, cold exposure, and a history of altitude sickness

■ Differential Diagnosis
  - Acute myocardial infarction
  - Exacerbation of preexisting heart condition
  - Pulmonary embolus
  - Pneumonia

■ Prevention & Treatment
  Prevention
  - Avoid exertion for 24 hours
  - Avoid alcohol for 24 hours
  - "Climb high, sleep low" (ie, sleep at a lower altitude than one climbs during the day)
  - Avoid dehydration
  - Take acetazolamide 250 mg every 8–12 hours, or dexamethasone 4 mg every 6–8 hours, the day before and 3–4 days at altitude
  Treatment
  - Descend to a lower altitude as soon as possible
  - Oxygen
  - Diuretics and morphine
  - Nifedipine 20 mg every 8 hours to lower pulmonary pressure
  - Phentolamine IV
  - Hyperbaric pressure bag

■ Pearl

When individuals with signs of acute mountain sickness (ie, malaise, headache, anorexia, and disturbed sleep) develop a dry cough, high-altitude pulmonary edema is imminent and preventive measures should be taken immediately.

Reference

Hultgren HN: High altitude pulmonary edema: Current concepts. Annu Rev Med 1996;47:267.

High-Output Heart Failure

- ■ Essentials of Diagnosis
  - • Symptoms and signs of congestive heart failure
  - • Echocardiographic or right-heart catheterization evidence of high cardiac output and normal systolic function
  - • Presence of a stimulus for high cardiac demands (eg, severe anemia, thyrotoxicosis, Paget disease, arteriovenous fistula, post liver transplantation, beriberi)

- ■ Differential Diagnosis
  - • Diastolic heart failure: normal systolic function, but low cardiac output
  - • Systolic dysfunction heart failure
  - • Fluid overload, usually iatrogenic

- ■ Treatment
  - • Eliminate the underlying cause
  - • Give diuretics to relieve congestion

- ■ Pearl

Bounding pulses with a wide pulse pressure are uncommon in systolic or diastolic heart failure unless severe aortic regurgitation is present.

Reference

Pfitzmann R et al: Liver transplantation for treatment of intrahepatic Osler's disease: First experiences. Transplantation 2001;72:237.

Hypertrophic Cardiomyopathies

- **Essentials of Diagnosis**
  - Dyspnea
  - Systolic ejection murmur with characteristic changes during bed-side maneuvers
  - Markedly asymmetric left ventricular hypertrophy on echocardiogram
  - Normal or hyperkinetic left ventricular systolic function

- **Differential Diagnosis**
  - Left ventricular hypertrophy secondary to other conditions (ie, hypertension)
  - Aortic stenosis with marked left ventricular hypertrophy
  - Restrictive cardiomyopathy with hypertrophy, such as amyloidosis
  - Ischemic heart disease with compensatory septal hypertrophy
  - Athlete's heart

- **Treatment**
  - Medical therapy: beta-blockers, calcium channel blockers, antibiotic prophylaxis for endocarditis, antiarrhythmics
  - Surgical therapy: septal myectomy to relieve left ventricular outflow tract obstruction; mitral valve replacement in selected cases
  - Other therapy: intracoronary ethanol septal ablation, pacemaker to set atrioventricular delay to minimize left ventricular outflow tract gradient, automatic implantable cardioverter-defibrillator

- **Pearl**

The Brockenbrough phenomenon refers to an analysis of the arterial pulse during cardiac catheterization. Usually in the beat after a premature ventricular contraction, the arterial pulse pressure is increased compared with the beat preceding the ectopic beat. This is true in a fixed obstruction to the left ventricle, such as aortic stenosis, as well. However, in hypertrophic cardiomyopathy, the pulse pressure is narrower because the increased left ventricular volume after the ectopic beat augments contractibility via the Frank-Starling mechanism, resulting in greater obstruction in left ventricular outflow, reduced stroke volume, and hence reduced pulse pressure. This phenomenon best illustrates the hemodynamic difference between a fixed obstruction (eg, aortic stenosis) and a dynamic one (ie, hypertrophic cardiomyopathy).

Reference

Elliott PM et al: Relation between severity of left-ventricular hypertrophy and prognosis in patients with hypertrophic cardiomyopathy. Lancet 2001;357:420.

Noncardiogenic Pulmonary Edema (Adult Respiratory Distress Syndrome; ARDS)

- ■ **Essentials of Diagnosis**
  - Bilateral diffuse alveolar infiltrates are present with severe hypoxemia
  - Pulmonary capillary wedge pressure (PCWP) is less than 18 mm Hg
  - ARDS represents the most serious form of acute lung injury and is defined by arterial PO_2/inspired oxygen concentration (PaO_2/FiO_2) of 200 mm Hg or less
  - ARDS may be a manifestation of several conditions, such as sepsis, aspiration, hypertransfusion, toxic inhalation, severe nonthoracic trauma, and cardiopulmonary bypass
  - Other incompletely understood causes include high-altitude pulmonary edema, neurogenic pulmonary edema, narcotic overdose, eclampsia, and cardioversion

- ■ **Differential Diagnosis**
  - Cardiogenic pulmonary edema (PCWP is typically >18 mm Hg)
  - Lymphangitic carcinomatosis (although PCWP is <18 mm Hg)
  - Unilateral pulmonary edema following evacuation of large pleural effusion (PCWP is normal)

- ■ **Treatment**
  - Treat the underlying cause if possible
  - Give supplemental oxygen and noninvasive ventilatory support in early stages of acute lung injury
  - Give mechanical ventilatory support with positive end-expiratory pressure and low tidal volumes (6–10 mL/kg) in established ARDS

- ■ **Pearl**

In young patients with ARDS and no obvious cause, do not forget narcotic overdose and concealed drug smuggling with elastic containers in the stomach or rectum.

Reference

Vincent JL et al: Epidemiology and outcome of acute respiratory failure in intensive care unit patients. Crit Care Med 2003;31:S296.

Pulmonary Edema, Acute

- **Essentials of Diagnosis**
  - Acute onset of profound dyspnea and orthopnea
  - Jugular venous distention, diffuse pulmonary rales, and tachycardia
  - Left ventricular systolic or diastolic dysfunction

- **Differential Diagnosis**
  - Pulmonary emboli
  - Bilateral pneumonia
  - ARDS

- **Treatment**
  - Oxygen, morphine sulfate
  - IV diuretics
  - IV catecholamines
  - IV phosphodiesterase inhibitors
  - IV vasodilators (eg, nitrates, nitroprusside, enalaprilat, hydralazine)
  - IV b-type natriuretic peptide

- **Pearl**

The most dramatic cases of acute pulmonary edema are often due to sudden disruption of the mitral valve apparatus, resulting in torrential mitral regurgitation. A history of acute myocardial infarction, uncontrolled hypertension, or symptoms of infective endocarditis may point to the etiology of sudden mitral valve failure.

Reference

Poole-Wilson PA, Xue SR: New therapies for the management of acute heart failure. Curr Cardiol Rep 2003;5:229.

Pulmonary Hypertension, Primary

- **Essentials of Diagnosis**
  - A rare disorder mostly seen in young women
  - No evidence of either lung or heart disease
  - Dyspnea, malaise, chest pain, or exertional syncope
  - Right ventricular lift
  - Increased intensity of the pulmonic component of the second heart sound
  - Elevated jugular *a* waves
  - ECG evidence of right ventricular hypertrophy
  - Elevated pulmonary artery pressures by Doppler echocardiography or cardiac catheterization

- **Differential Diagnosis**
  - Mitral stenosis
  - Sleep apnea
  - Chronic pulmonary embolism
  - Autoimmune diseases such as scleroderma
  - Left ventricular failure
  - Congenital heart disease
  - Cirrhosis of the liver with portopulmonary hypertension
  - Pulmonary veno-occlusive disease

- **Treatment**
  - Oxygen supplementation for severe right-heart failure with hypoxia at rest (some patients may have exercise-related hypoxia)
  - Continuous IV prostacyclin improves survival
  - Empiric anticoagulation may confer survival benefit
  - Bosentan (oral endothelin antagonist) may be useful in mild to moderate pulmonary hypertension
  - Other oral vasodilators have unpredictable and uncertain efficacy (eg, calcium channel blockers)
  - Heart-lung transplantation may be needed in eligible patients

- **Pearl**

Exclude mitral stenosis before diagnosing primary pulmonary hypertension.

Reference

Gaine SP et al: Primary pulmonary hypertension. Lancet 1998;352:719.

Myocarditis/Pericarditis

Acquired Immunodeficiency Syndrome (AIDS) & the Heart

- **Essentials of Diagnosis**
  - Pericardial effusion
  - Lymphocytic interstitial myocarditis
  - Dilated cardiomyopathy and left ventricular systolic dysfunction
  - Infective endocarditis
  - Myocardial Kaposi sarcoma and B-cell immunoblastic lymphoma
  - Pulmonary hypertension secondary to multiple pulmonary infarctions, or primary pulmonary hypertension
  - Accelerated atherosclerosis as a consequence of longer survival and the use of antiretroviral agents

- **Differential Diagnosis**
  - Idiopathic dilated cardiomyopathy
  - Heart failure secondary to foscarnet used for cytomegalovirus infection
  - Dilated cardiomyopathy secondary to interferon-alfa used to treat Kaposi sarcoma
  - Other causes of pericardial effusion

- **Treatment**
  - Management of hyperlipidemia
  - Management of heart failure similar to that for dilated cardiomyopathy
  - Pericardiocentesis, pericardial window, biopsy as needed
  - Therapy for infections
  - Chemotherapy for Kaposi sarcoma and lymphoma

- **Pearl**

Human immunodeficiency virus (HIV) is becoming a chronic disease. Treat risk factors as in the non–HIV-infected population.

Reference

Barbaro G: Cardiovascular manifestations of HIV infection. Circulation 2002;106:1420.

Cardiac Tamponade

- ■ Essentials of Diagnosis
  - Increased jugular venous pressure with an obliterated y descent
  - Pulsus paradoxus
  - Echocardiographic evidence of right atrial and ventricular collapse
  - Equal diastolic pressures in all 4 cardiac chambers

- ■ Differential Diagnosis
  - Cardiogenic shock
  - Severe obstructive airway disease
  - Congestive heart failure
  - Pulmonary embolus
  - Constrictive pericarditis
  - Tension pneumothorax

- ■ Treatment
  - Immediate pericardial fluid drainage
  - Intravenous fluids until drainage can be accomplished
  - In selected cases, surgical drainage is required with creation of a pericardial to pleural opening. A percutaneous balloon technique for creating a pleuropericardial opening has been described.

- ■ Pearl

In patients who become hypotensive during dialysis, low-pressure cardiac tamponade should be considered. These patients have small to moderate pericardial effusions that do not cause tamponade under normal conditions, but when intravascular depletion occurs and right-heart pressures decrease, intrapericardial pressure may exceed cardiac pressures, causing tamponade.

Reference

Lindenberger M et al: Pericardiocentesis guided by 2-D echocardiography: The method of choice for treatment of pericardial effusion. J Intern Med 2003;253:411.

Lyme Carditis

- **Essentials of Diagnosis**
  - Infectious disease is caused by *Borrelia burgdorferi*, a tick-borne spirochete
  - Initial manifestations include myalgias, arthralgia, fever, headache, and a skin rash called erythema migrans
  - 10% of infected patients develop symptoms from transient cardiac involvement weeks to months after initial presentation
  - The most common manifestation is conduction abnormality in the form of varying degrees of atrioventricular block
  - Syncope due to complete heart block is common
  - Diffuse ST-segment and T-wave changes and asymptomatic left ventricular dysfunction may be found, but congestive heart failure is rare

- **Differential Diagnosis**
  - Myocarditis due to other infectious agents
  - Intrinsic conduction system disease

- **Treatment**
  - Antibiotic therapy with penicillin or doxycycline is recommended
  - Cardiac monitoring is needed for identification of complete heart block
  - Temporary transvenous pacemaker may be required
  - Glucocorticoids may be of benefit if there is no improvement with antimicrobial therapy

- **Pearl**

Conduction system abnormalities in Lyme disease are usually transient, but a temporary pacemaker may be needed for a week or longer.

Reference

Donta ST: Late and chronic Lyme disease. Med Clin North Am 2002;86:341.

Myocarditis

- **Essentials of Diagnosis**
  - Focal or diffuse inflammation of the myocardium due to various infections, toxins, drugs, or immunologic reactions
  - Viral infection, particularly with coxsackie viruses, is the most common cause
  - Other infectious causes include HIV infection, Lyme disease, Rocky Mountain spotted fever, trichinosis, toxoplasmosis, and acute rheumatic fever
  - New congestive heart failure with an antecedent viral syndrome
  - Elevated erythrocyte sedimentation rate or cardiac biomarkers
  - Electrocardiogram (ECG) shows sinus tachycardia, nonspecific ST-T changes, atrial or ventricular arrhythmias, or conduction abnormalities
  - Echocardiogram demonstrates chamber enlargement, wall motion abnormalities, systolic or diastolic dysfunction, or mural thrombi
  - Routine endomyocardial biopsy is not recommended because inflammatory changes are often focal and nonspecific. When positive, the changes include inflammatory infiltrate with adjacent myocyte injury.

- **Differential Diagnosis**
  - Acute myocardial ischemia or infarction due to coronary artery disease
  - Pneumonia
  - Congestive heart failure due to other causes

- **Treatment**
  - Strict bed rest (animal models show increased intensity of inflammation, morbidity, and mortality with exercise)
  - Specific antimicrobial treatment if an infectious agent is identified
  - Immunosuppressive therapy is generally not helpful except in giant-cell myocarditis and immune diseases such as systemic lupus erythematosus
  - Appropriate treatment of systolic dysfunction (angiotensin-converting enzyme inhibitors, beta-blockers, digoxin, spironolactone, and diuretics)
  - Cardiac transplantation

- **Pearl**

Remember the "rule of thirds" for patients with viral myocarditis: One third return to normal, one third have stable left ventricular dysfunction, and one third have a rapidly deteriorating course.

Reference

Pisani B et al: Inflammatory myocardial diseases and cardiomyopathies. Am J Med 1997;102:459.

Pericardial Effusion

- **Essentials of Diagnosis**
  - Echocardiographic demonstration of pericardial fluid

- **Differential Diagnosis**
  - Pericardial fat is indistinguishable on echocardiogram
  - Chylous pericardial fluid may be present from thoracic duct obstruction

- **Treatment**
  - Small: treat underlying cause (eg, hypothyroidism)
  - Moderate: monitor carefully during specific causal therapy
  - Large: risk of tamponade is high; drainage is recommended
  - Moderate to large: with signs of hemodynamic compromise on echocardiography, but no clinical tamponade, drainage is recommended

- **Pearl**

Large pericardial effusions can result in high, then low P-QRS-T voltage amplitude on every other beat (electrical alternans) because of a swinging motion of the heart at half the heart rate frequency.

Reference

Tsang TS et al: Outcomes of clinically significant idiopathic pericardial effusion requiring intervention. Am J Cardiol 2002;91:704.

Pericarditis, Acute

- **Essentials of Diagnosis**
  - Central chest pain aggravated by coughing, inspiration, or recumbency
  - Pericardial friction rub on auscultation
  - Characteristic ECG changes

- **Differential Diagnosis**
  - Acute myocardial infarction
  - Aortic dissection
  - Pulmonary embolus
  - Pneumothorax
  - Pneumonia

- **Treatment**
  - Treat underlying cause (eg, uremia)
  - Nonsteroidal anti-inflammatory agents
  - Steroids if unresponsive to nonsteroidal anti-inflammatories
  - Colchicine for recurrent pericarditis
  - Pericardiectomy in rare cases

- **Pearl**

An ECG T-wave height to ST-height ratio in V6 of 4 or higher suggests early repolarization, whereas a ratio of less than 4 suggests pericarditis.

Reference

Marinella MA: Electrocardiographic manifestations and differential diagnosis of acute pericarditis. Am Fam Physician 1998;57:699.

Pericarditis, Constrictive

- ■ Essentials of Diagnosis
  - Markedly elevated jugular venous pressure with accentuated x and y descents and Kussmaul sign
  - Pericardial knock on auscultation
  - Magnetic resonance, computed tomography, or echocardiographic imaging showing a thickened pericardium

- ■ Differential Diagnosis
  - Cardiac tamponade
  - Restrictive cardiomyopathy
  - Right-heart failure
  - Cirrhosis with ascites
  - Malabsorption syndrome

- ■ Treatment
  - Surgical pericardiectomy

- ■ Pearl

A low cardiac output state may occur after surgery because of myocardial atrophy from long-term compression and may require prolonged pressor therapy until myocardial function can recover.

Reference

Myers RB, Spodick DH: Constrictive pericarditis: Clinical and pathophysiologic characteristics. Am Heart J 1999;138:219.

Pericarditis, Effusive-Constrictive

- **Essentials of Diagnosis**
  - Echocardiographic demonstration of pericardial fluid with strands and constrictive physiology
  - Persistence of elevated intracardiac filling pressures following pericardicentesis with constrictive features
  - Common causes are uremia, malignancy, radiation, and tuberculosis

- **Differential Diagnosis**
  - Cardiac tamponade
  - Constrictive pericarditis
  - Restrictive cardiomyopathy with incidental pericardial effusion

- **Treatment**
  - Treat underlying cause if known
  - Pericardial resection is often required

- **Pearl**

Pericardial effusion alone is usually not associated with Kussmaul sign. Suspect effusive-constrictive pericarditis when these 2 findings occur together.

Reference

Hoit BD: Management of effusive and constrictive pericardial heart disease. Circulation 2002;105:2939.

Hypertension

Hypertension, Gestational

- **Essentials of Diagnosis**
  - Hypertension occurs after 20 weeks of gestation or up to 6 weeks postpartum in previously normotensive women
  - Usually diagnosed after a rise in blood pressure of 30/15 mm Hg or more, to a level above 140/90 mm Hg
  - May progress to preeclampsia when complicated by proteinuria, edema, or hematologic or hepatic abnormalities
  - May progress to cerebral symptoms, leading to convulsions
  - Women with hypertension predating pregnancy have a higher incidence of preeclampsia
  - Although the cause is unknown, it occurs more frequently in primigravidas and in subsequent pregnancies with a different father

- **Differential Diagnosis**
  - Chronic hypertension
  - Unclassified hypertension when blood pressure status before conception and during first trimester is unknown

- **Treatment**
  - Bed rest and methyldopa are the primary treatments
  - Hydralazine, nifedipine, and labetalol may be used in succession for severe hypertension
  - Angiotensin-converting enzyme inhibitors and angiotensin-receptor blockers are contraindicated
  - For intrapartum management, intravenous (IV) magnesium is used to prevent progression of preeclampsia to seizures

- **Pearl**

Excessive magnesium can cause respiratory depression. A bedside early warning sign of overdose is loss of deep tendon reflexes.

Reference

Borghi C et al: The treatment of hypertension in pregnancy. J Hypertens 2002;20(suppl 2):S52.

Hypertension, Renovascular

- ■ Essentials of Diagnosis
  - Severe hypertension occurring before age 25 or after age 55 years
  - Abdominal or flank systolic and diastolic bruits, or evidence of peripheral vascular disease
  - Unilateral small kidney on any imaging study
  - Hypertension resistant to 3 medications
  - Worsening of renal function after an angiotensin-converting enzyme inhibitor
  - Elevated plasma renin activity with or without captopril administration
  - Imaging evidence of renal artery occlusive disease

- ■ Differential Diagnosis
  - Essential hypertension
  - Renal parenchymal disease
  - Other causes of secondary hypertension

- ■ Treatment
  - Pharmacologic therapy if hypertension is mild or readily controlled
  - Percutaneous angioplasty with or without stenting
  - Surgical repair or nephrectomy

- ■ Pearl

One in 5 patients with significant renal artery stenosis will present with flash pulmonary edema not due to ischemic heart disease. They almost always have bilateral renal artery stenosis or 1 functioning kidney.

Reference

Safian RD, Textor SC: Renal artery stenosis. N Engl J Med 2001;344:431.

Hypertension, Systemic

- **Essentials of Diagnosis**
  - Diastolic pressure greater than 90 mm Hg, systolic pressure greater than 140 mm Hg, or both, on 3 separate occasions
  - In diabetic patients, diastolic pressure greater than 80 mm Hg, systolic pressure greater than 130 mm Hg, or both, on 3 separate occasions

- **Differential Diagnosis**
  - Pseudo- or white-coat hypertension
  - High-output state (eg, marked aortic regurgitation)
  - Secondary causes: steroid therapy (eg, oral contraceptives), pheochromocytoma, coarctation of the aorta, renal artery stenosis, Cushing syndrome, primary hyperaldosteronism, chronic alcohol use

- **Treatment**
  - Nonpharmacologic: lose weight, get regular exercise, reduce alcohol consumption, restrict sodium intake, reduce stress levels
  - Pharmacologic: alpha-adrenergic blockers, beta-adrenergic blockers, angiotensin-converting enzyme inhibitors, angiotensin-receptor blockers, calcium channel blockers, diuretics, central nervous system agents, and direct peripheral vasodilators

- **Pearl**

Orthostatic hypotension in a patient with hypertension suggests pheochromocytoma.

Reference

MacMahon S: Blood pressure and the risk of cardiovascular disease. N Engl J Med 2000;342:50.

Hypertensive Emergencies

- **Essentials of Diagnosis**
  - Blood pressure greater than 220/120 mm Hg and
  - Symptoms and signs of encephalopathy, acute myocardial ischemia, stroke, pulmonary edema, or aortic dissection

- **Differential Diagnosis**
  - Increased intracranial pressure—lowering blood pressure contraindicated
  - Acute drug-induced pressure elevation (eg, cocaine)

- **Treatment**
  - Nitroprusside 0.25–10 μg/kg/min
  - Fenoldopam 0.1 μg/kg/min, increase by 0.05 μg/kg/min
  - Labetalol 20–40 mg IV every 10 minutes to 300 mg
  - Esmolol 500 μg/kg over 1 minute, then 25–200 μg/kg/min
  - Clonidine 0.1–0.2 mg orally, 0.05–0.1 mg every hour to 0.8 mg
  - Captopril 6.24–50 mg orally every 6–8 hours

- **Pearl**

Oral immediate-release nifedipine can cause unpredictable hypotension and should not be used.

Reference

Lip GYH et al: Survival and prognosis of 315 patients with malignant-phase hypertension. J Hypertens 1995;13:915.

Hypertensive Nephrosclerosis

- Essentials of Diagnosis
  - Chronic systemic hypertension before the onset of proteinuria
  - Declining renal function, proteinuria
  - Renal biopsy evidence of hyaline arteriolar sclerosis (afferent), myointimal hypertrophy/hyperplasia, and fibrinoid necrosis

- Differential Diagnosis
  - Because renal biopsy is rarely performed, hypertensive nephrosclerosis is usually a diagnosis of exclusion
  - Parenchymal renal disease
  - Renovascular hypertension with renal insufficiency

- Treatment
  - 24-hour blood pressure less than 130/85 mm Hg with multiple drugs as necessary
  - Sodium restriction and diuretics
  - Angiotensin-converting enzyme inhibitors or angiotensin-receptor blockers

- Pearl

Hypertensive nephrosclerosis is most common in African-American males, in whom beta-blockers and angiotensin-converting enzyme inhibitors are less effective than calcium blockers and diuretics.

Reference

Moore MA et al: Current strategies for management of hypertensive renal disease. Arch Intern Med 1999;159:23.

Pheochromocytoma

- ■ Essentials of Diagnosis
  - • Biochemical evidence of excess catecholamines
  - • Adrenal tumor or tumor along the sympathetic chain (paraganglioma)
  - • Headache, palpitations, and sweating in conjunction with either hypertension (may be paroxysmal) or orthostatic hypotension
  - • Pressor response to anesthesia induction or to antihypertensive or sympathomimetic drugs

- ■ Differential Diagnosis
  - • Other causes of hypertension, headaches, palpitations, and orthostatic hypotension

- ■ Treatment
  - • Surgical removal of the catecholamine-producing tumor(s)
  - • Preoperative alpha- and beta-blockade

- ■ Pearl

Suspect pheochromocytoma in any patient who develops a sudden elevation in blood pressure during anesthesia induction.

Reference

Plouin P et al: Factors associated with perioperative morbidity and mortality in patients with pheochromocytoma: Analysis of 165 operations at a single center. J Clin Endocrinol Metab 2001;86:1480.

Resistant or Refractory Hypertension

- **Essentials of Diagnosis**
  - Blood pressure greater than 140/90 mm Hg in patients adhering to a triple-drug regimen (including a diuretic) at near-maximal doses
  - In older patients, systolic blood pressure greater than 160 mm Hg despite adequate triple-drug therapy

- **Differential Diagnosis**
  - Inaccurate blood pressure measurement (eg, cuff too small)
  - Stimulant exposure (eg, nasal sprays, diet pills, alcohol)
  - Aggravating medical conditions (eg, sleep apnea)
  - Secondary hypertension (eg, renal artery stenosis)

- **Treatment**
  - Intensify lifestyle modifications (eg, low-salt diet, exercise)
  - Maximize medications, especially diuretics
  - Try to use the most efficacious combinations of drugs first (eg, a diuretic, an angiotensin-converting enzyme inhibitor, and a calcium channel blocker), then add either a beta-blocker or a central alpha-2-receptor agonist such as clonidine, or a combined adrenergic inhibitor such as labetalol

- **Pearl**

Twenty-four–hour ambulatory blood pressure measurements may be useful to tailor drug administration times to your patient's blood pressure rhythms.

Reference

Oparil S et al: Managing the patient with hard to control hypertension. Am Fam Physician 1998;57:1007.

7

Congenital Heart Disease

Atrial Septal Defect (ASD)

- ■ Essentials of Diagnosis
  - A widely fixed split second heart sound and a mid-systolic murmur are characteristic. If the shunt is large, a mid-diastolic rumble of relative tricuspid stenosis may be audible at the lower left sternal border.
  - Incomplete right bundle branch block with vertical QRS axis (ostium secundum ASD) and superior axis (ostium primum ASD) on electrocardiography (ECG)
  - Prominent pulmonary arteries and right ventricular enlargement (decreased retrosternal air space) on chest radiograph; increased pulmonary vascular markings
  - Right ventricular dilatation, increased pulmonary artery flow velocity, and left-to-right atrial shunt by Doppler echocardiography
  - Oxygen step-up within the right atrium; right-sided catheter can pass into the left atrium across the defect

- ■ Differential Diagnosis
  - Other causes of exertional dyspnea, of atrial arrhythmias, of right ventricular failure, and of a mid-systolic murmur (eg, pulmonic stenosis)
  - The wide fixed split second heart sound can be mimicked by complete right bundle branch block, pericardial knock, and a late systolic click
  - Other causes of pulmonary hypertension

- ■ Treatment
  - Surgical correction is recommended for a left-to-right shunt greater than 1.5:1.0.
  - Smaller shunts can be closed if paradoxical systemic embolization cannot be controlled by other means, such as anticoagulation
  - Small ostium secundum defects with adequate membranous tissue rims can be closed with a percutaneously delivered mechanical closure device; experience with such devices is increasing
  - Pulmonary hypertension and older age increase the risk of surgical closure. Surgery is relatively contraindicated when pulmonary vascular resistance is greater than $10–15 \ U/m^2$.

- ■ Pearl

Sinus venosus defects often cause ectopic atrial rhythm with a superior P-wave axis.

Reference

Hung J et al: Closure of patent foramen ovale for paradoxical emboli: Intermediate term risk of recurrent neurological events following transcatheter device placement. J Am Coll Cardiol 2000;35:1311.

Atrioventricular Canal Defects

- ■ Essentials of Diagnosis
  - • Infant with congestive heart failure
  - • Physical findings include ASD plus mitral regurgitation
  - • Cardiac imaging shows a common atrioventricular (AV) valve annulus, 1 or more abnormal AV valves, and defects at the atrial or the ventricular level that can be detected in utero

- ■ Differential Diagnosis
  - • Secundum ASD with mitral regurgitation due to rheumatic disease or prolapse
  - • Ventricular septal defect
  - • Other causes of heart failure

- ■ Treatment
  - • Complete surgical repair is needed
  - • Mitral regurgitation may require repeat operation

- ■ Pearl

In the right anterior oblique view on left ventricular angiography, the change in AV valve position makes the inlet portion of the ventricular septum appear scooped out and the outflow tract elongated. This results in a "goose-neck" appearance, where the aortic sinuses of Valsalva are the head, the elongated outflow tract is the neck, and the left ventricle is the body.

Reference

Acar P et al: Three-dimensional echocardiographic analysis of valve anatomy as a determinant of mitral regurgitation after surgery for atrioventricular septal defects. Am J Cardiol 1999;83:745.

Coarctation of the Aorta

- **Essentials of Diagnosis**
  - Elevated systolic blood pressure in the upper extremities (always in right arm); normal systolic blood pressure in lower extremities (and often in left arm)
  - Radial-femoral pulse delay
  - Left ventricular hypertrophy, left ventricular prominence, "3" sign, rib-notching on chest radiograph
  - Coarctation visible by imaging
  - Distal aortic pressure drop by Doppler echocardiography or catheterization

- **Differential Diagnosis**
  - Other causes of systemic hypertension
  - Aortoiliac disease

- **Treatment**
  - Antibiotic prophylaxis should be given for infective endocarditis
  - Surgical correction is indicated for significant obstruction: peak systolic gradient greater than 10 mm Hg
  - One third of patients operated on after age 14 years will require therapy for persistent hypertension
  - Recurrent coarctation after surgical correction can usually be treated with balloon angioplasty with or without a stent

- **Pearl**

Associated conditions include bicuspid aortic valve, congenital mitral valve disease, and aneurysms of the circle of Willis.

Reference

Kaemmerer H et al: Arterial hypertension in adults after surgical treatment of aortic coarctation. Thorac Cardiovasc Surg 1998;46:121.

Congenitally Corrected Transposition of the Great Arteries

- ■ Essentials of Diagnosis
  - Prominent left parasternal impulse, soft first heart sound, accentuated second heart sound with soft or inaudible pulmonic component
  - P-R prolongation, variable degrees of AV block, Q waves in right precordial leads with absence in left precordial leads on ECG
  - Absence of left-sided aortic knob on chest radiograph
  - Rightward and posterior pulmonary artery with leftward and anterior aorta; apical displacement of right-sided AV valve; coarsely trabeculated left-sided systemic ventricle with moderator band (the morphologic right ventricle) on cardiac imaging

- ■ Differential Diagnosis
  - Other causes of complete heart block
  - Other causes of heart failure

- ■ Treatment
  - Pacemaker for heart block
  - Surgery for associated lesions when indicated: pulmonic stenosis; ventricular septal defect; tricuspid valve repair or replacement
  - Cardiac transplantation

- ■ Pearl

Tricuspid valve abnormalities (Ebstein-like deformities) reduce the chance for survival because the systemic ventricle (anatomic right ventricle) is less tolerant of AV valve regurgitation (tricuspid valve) than the anatomic left ventricle, resulting in a vicious cycle of more regurgitation and more heart failure.

Reference

Graham TP Jr et al: Long-term outcome in congenitally corrected transposition of the great arteries: A multi-institutional study. J Am Coll Cardiol 2000;36:255.

Ebstein Anomaly

- ■ Essentials of Diagnosis
  - • History of dyspnea, atypical chest pain, or intermittent cyanosis
  - • Palpitations associated with supraventricular arrhythmias and pre-excitation syndrome
  - • Right parasternal lift, widely split first heart sound, systolic clicks, and systolic murmur of tricuspid regurgitation (without inspiratory accentuation)
  - • Right atrial enlargement, right ventricular conduction defect of right bundle branch block type, posteriorly directed delta waves with accessory pathway by ECG; frequent first-degree AV block
  - • Normal or reduced pulmonary vascularity without pulmonary artery enlargement, right atrial enlargement, normal left-sided cardiac silhouette on chest radiograph
  - • Apical displacement of septal tricuspid valve leaflet, variable degrees of tricuspid regurgitation originating from apical portion of right ventricle, and enlarged right atrium on echocardiography

- ■ Differential Diagnosis
  - • Other causes of tricuspid regurgitation
  - • Other causes of exertional dyspnea, chest pressure, and intermittent cyanosis
  - • Other causes of supraventricular arrhythmias
  - • Other causes of congestive heart failure

- ■ Treatment
  - • Catheter ablation of bypass tracts and other foci of supraventricular arrhythmia
  - • Tricuspid valve repair or replacement
  - • Fontan procedure (connection of systemic venous drainage to the pulmonary artery)

- ■ Pearl

ASD frequently coexists with Ebstein anomaly and explains the intermittent cyanosis often observed when right atrial pressures rise.

Reference

DiRusso GB et al: Ebstein's anomaly: Indications for repair and surgical technique. In: Spray TL et al: Seminars in Thoracic and Cardiovascular Surgery, Pediatric Cardiac Surgery Annual 1999. WB Saunders, 1999.

Eisenmenger Syndrome

- **Essentials of Diagnosis**
  - History of murmur or cyanosis in infancy; symptoms of dyspnea and exercise intolerance since childhood
  - Hemoptysis, chest pain, and syncope in the adult
  - Clubbing, cyanosis, and prominent pulmonic component of the second heart sound
  - Compensatory erythrocytosis, iron deficiency, and hyperuricemia
  - Right ventricular hypertrophy; large central pulmonary arteries with peripheral pruning on chest radiograph
  - Severe right ventricular hypertrophy and right atrial enlargement, elevated pulmonary artery pressures, and pulmonary insufficiency on Doppler echocardiography
  - Detection of a bidirectional shunt by echocardiography or cardiac catheterization

- **Differential Diagnosis**
  - Pulmonary emboli
  - Other causes of hemoptysis, chest pain, and syncope
  - Other causes of cyanosis

- **Treatment**
  - Once pulmonary vascular resistance is fixed (no response to oxygen or nitrous oxide inhalation), surgical correction of the underlying communication between the right and left heart is contra-indicated
  - Phlebotomy when hematocrit is greater than 65%
  - Counseling regarding contraception in women of reproductive age because pregnancy is extremely dangerous
  - Cardiac transplantation

- **Pearl**

Transient bacteremias can result in brain abscess because of right-to-left shunting before the pulmonary circulation, which normally filters bacteria.

Reference

Hopkins WE: Severe pulmonary hypertension in congenital heart disease: A review of Eisenmenger syndrome. Curr Opin Cardiol 1995;10:517.

Kawasaki Disease

- **Essentials of Diagnosis**
  - Acute vasculitis of unknown etiology that occurs mostly in infants and children
  - Fever lasting 5 or more days
  - Bilateral nonexudative conjunctival injection
  - Injected lips or pharynx, or "strawberry tongue"
  - Acute nonsuppurative cervical lymphadenopathy
  - Erythema of the palms and soles, or polymorphous exanthem
  - Exclusion of common bacterial and viral infections
  - Coronary artery aneurysms, myocarditis, and valve regurgitation

- **Differential Diagnosis**
  - Streptococcal and staphylococcal infections
  - Measles, enterovirus, and adenovirus infections
  - Systemic allergic reactions to medications

- **Treatment**
  - Aspirin 100 mg/kg/d in 4 divided doses and, once fever subsides, 3–5 mg/kg/d for 6–8 weeks
  - Intravenous gamma globulin 2 g/kg in a single infusion, preferably within 10 days of onset of symptoms
  - Coronary stenosis may be treated with bypass surgery
  - If coronary aneurysms develop, long-term antiplatelet therapy with aspirin or clopidogrel
  - Longitudinal follow-up with echocardiogram for coronary aneurysms

- **Pearl**

Although Kawasaki disease was first described in Japan and was most prevalent there, it is now seen worldwide. However, the incidence in Asians is 5–10 times that in Caucasians.

Reference

Sundel RP: Update on the treatment of Kawasaki disease in childhood. Curr Rheumatol Rep 2002;4:474.

Partial Anomalous Pulmonary Venous Connection

- ■ Essentials of Diagnosis
  - • Young adult with dyspnea, recurrent respiratory infections, hemoptysis, and palpitations
  - • Physical findings of ASD: right ventricular heave, systolic ejection murmur at the left sternal border, wide fixed split of second heart sound, and a diastolic flow rumble over the tricuspid area
  - • Incomplete right bundle branch block on ECG
  - • Pulmonary vascular congestion, enlarged right heart, and occasionally evidence of the anomalous vein on chest radiograph
  - • Cardiac imaging evidence of anomalous pulmonary venous connection and ASD in many patients

- ■ Differential Diagnosis
  - • ASD
  - • Right-heart failure from other causes
  - • Pulmonary hypertension from other causes

- ■ Treatment
  - • Surgical correction for shunts greater than 2:1 and symptoms
  - • Supportive care in nonsurgical cases for heart failure and arrhythmias

- ■ Pearl

When the right pulmonary veins form 1 trunk connected to the inferior vena cava at the level of the diaphragm, the resulting shadow from this anomalous trunk resembles a curved sword on the plain radiograph of the chest and has been called the "scimitar syndrome."

Reference

Wong ML et al: Echocardiographic evaluation of partial anomalous pulmonary venous drainage. J Am Coll Cardiol 1995;26:503.

Patent Ductus Arteriosus

- Essentials of Diagnosis
  - Continuous machinery-like murmur, loudest below the left clavicle
  - Left ventricular hypertrophy
  - Pulmonary plethora, left atrial and ventricular enlargement; in older adults, calcification of the ductus on chest radiograph
  - Left atrial and ventricular dilatation with normal right-heart chambers on echocardiography
  - Continuous high-velocity color Doppler jet with retrograde flow along lateral wall of main pulmonary artery near left branch

- Differential Diagnosis
  - Other causes of exertional dyspnea, chest pain, and palpitations
  - Other causes of left-heart dilatation and failure
  - The characteristic continuous murmur can be mimicked by aortic stenosis with regurgitation, mitral stenosis with regurgitation, and ventricular septal defect with aortic regurgitation

- Treatment
  - Antibiotic prophylaxis is needed for infective endocarditis
  - Surgical closure should be done for left-to-right shunts greater than 2:1
  - Surgical risk is elevated with pulmonary vascular resistance greater than 10 U/m^2 and older age
  - Percutaneous coil occlusion of the duct is often feasible and reduces the risk of endocarditis

- Pearl

When pulmonary vascular resistance rises and reverses the shunt (right to left), differential cyanosis develops. Because the duct usually inserts below the left subclavian artery in adults, the feet are cyanotic, but not the hands.

Reference

Harrison DA et al: Percutaneous catheter closure of the persistently patent ductus arteriosus in the adult. Am J Cardiol 1996;77:1094.

Patent Foramen Ovale/Atrial Septal Aneurysm

- ### Essentials of Diagnosis
  - Cryptogenic stroke due to paradoxical embolus
  - Doppler echocardiographic evidence of patent foramen ovale
  - Combination of patent foramen ovale and atrial septal aneurysm carries the highest risk of recurrent stroke; atrial septal aneurysm alone is not associated with recurrent stroke

- ### Differential Diagnosis
  - ASD
  - Bowed, hypermobile, but intact atrial septum without aneurysm
  - Other causes of cryptogenic stroke, such as mitral valve prolapse, left atrial myxoma, and infective endocarditis

- ### Treatment
  Asymptomatic patients
  - No specific treatment is warranted
  Symptomatic patients have 4 options
  - Antiplatelet drugs such as aspirin or clopidogrel
  - Anticoagulants such as warfarin
  - Percutaneous transcatheter closure devices
  - Surgical closure

- ### Pearl

  Younger patients without typical risk factors for stroke (diabetes, hypertension, atherosclerotic vascular disease) should always undergo transthoracic echocardiography with agitated saline contrast and the Valsalva maneuver to detect patent foramen ovale. If doubt exists, transesophageal echocardiography should be considered.

Reference

Mas JL et al: Recurrent cerebrovascular events associated with patent foramen ovale, atrial septal aneurysm or both. N Engl J Med 2001;345:1740.

Pulmonary Atresia with Intact Ventricular Septum

- ■ Essentials of Diagnosis
  - • History of cyanosis at birth, worsening at the time of ductal closure
  - • Single second heart sound; continuous murmur is rare
  - • Prominent left ventricular forces
  - • Oligemic lung fields, enlarged cardiac silhouette on chest radiograph
  - • ASD, small right ventricle, absent pulmonary valve; in adults, a palliative shunt or right ventricle to pulmonary artery conduit

- ■ Differential Diagnosis
  - • Tricuspid atresia
  - • Other causes of cyanosis

- ■ Treatment
  - • In the older child with an adequate size of the right ventricle, a right ventricle to main pulmonary artery conduit is placed (Rastelli procedure)
  - • In those with a rudimentary right ventricle, a Fontan procedure is done (cavocaval baffle to pulmonary artery connection)

- ■ Pearl

High pressure in the right ventricle may be partially decompressed through dilated coronary sinusoids into the left or right coronary artery. This phenomenon is inversely related to the severity of tricuspid regurgitation. After surgical decompression of the right ventricle by connecting it to the pulmonary circulation, coronary flow in the right ventricle is reversed, which can produce a coronary to right ventricle "steal," resulting in myocardial ischemia. If these right ventricular sinusoids are detected by angiography before surgery, a systemic to pulmonary artery shunt can be performed.

Reference

Gatzoulis MA et al: Definitive palliation with cavopulmonary or aortopulmonary shunts for adults with single ventricle physiology. Heart 2000;83:51.

Pulmonary Atresia with Ventricular Septal Defect

- ■ Essentials of Diagnosis
  - • DiGeorge syndrome in 40%
  - • Pulmonary blood flow entirely from patent ductus arteriosus or major aortopulmonary collateral arteries
  - • Infant with mild to profound cyanosis, depending on the amount of pulmonary blood flow
  - • Continuous murmurs over the thorax
  - • Congestive heart failure in 25%
  - • Right aortic arch in 50%
  - • Cardiac imaging evidence of the defect

- ■ Differential Diagnosis
  - • Tetralogy of Fallot
  - • Patent ductus arteriosus
  - • Truncus arteriosus
  - • Other causes of cyanosis and heart failure

- ■ Treatment
  - • Initial management is prostaglandin E_1 administration for those infants with ductal dependent pulmonary circulation
  - • Palliative shunts to increase pulmonary blood flow (eg, Blalock-Taussig)
  - • Surgical repair, which may include conduits
  - • Reoperation is often necessary to replace conduits or take down palliative shunts before corrective surgery

- ■ Pearl

Although the aortic valve is usually anatomically normal, significant aortic regurgitation occurs in about three quarters of patients with pulmonary atresia and ventricular septal defect.

Reference

Marelli AJ et al: Pulmonary atresia with ventricular septal defect in adults. Circulation 1994;89:243.

Sinus of Valsalva Aneurysm

- **Essentials of Diagnosis**
  - Diverticulum of a coronary sinus of the aortic valve
  - May rupture and create a fistula with another cardiac chamber, usually the right ventricle
  - May be associated with connective tissue diseases such as Marfan syndrome
  - May be associated with other congenital heart diseases, such as supracristal ventricular septal defect
  - May be acquired from a vasculitis such as syphilis

- **Differential Diagnosis**
  - Aortic dissection
  - Aortic regurgitation with aortic root dilatation
  - Aorta to pulmonary artery fistula (anterior-posterior window)
  - Ventricular septal defect
  - Coronary artery aneurysm with fistula to right heart
  - Rupture may simulate other causes of acute chest pain, or heart failure

- **Treatment**
  - Maintain forward circulation in acute rupture with vasodilator drugs such as nitroprusside or angiotensin-converting enzyme inhibitors
  - Close defect with percutaneous transcatheter device
  - Surgical repair may be needed
  - Unruptured aneurysm should be monitored and hypertension should be treated
  - Whether prophylactic therapy with vasodilators is beneficial is unknown

- **Pearl**

An unruptured sinus of Valsalva aneurysm may present as obstruction of the right ventricular outflow tract or the mitral valve.

Reference

Hijazi ZM: Ruptured sinus of Valsalva aneurysm: Management options. Catheter Cardiovasc Interv 2003;58:135.

Tetralogy of Fallot

- ### Essentials of Diagnosis
  - History of exercise intolerance and squatting during childhood
  - Central cyanosis, mildly prominent right ventricular impulse, murmur of pulmonic stenosis (with sufficient pulmonary blood flow), and absent pulmonic component of the second heart sound
  - Mild right ventricular hypertrophy; occasionally left ventricular hypertrophy
  - Chest radiograph shows classic boot-shaped heart (coeur en sabot) in severe cases without left-to-right shunt; left ventricular enlargement and post-stenotic pulmonary artery dilatation in milder cases; right-sided aortic arch in approximately 25% of patients
  - Echocardiogram shows right ventricular hypertrophy, overriding aorta, large perimembranous ventricular septal defect, and obstruction of the right ventricular outflow tract (subvalvular, valvular, supravalvular, or in the pulmonary arterial branches)
  - Gradient across pulmonary outflow tract, normal pulmonary artery pressures, equalization of right and left ventricular pressures on catheterization
  - Possibly anomalous branches of right coronary artery crossing right ventricular outflow tract on coronary angiography

- ### Differential Diagnosis
  - Truncus arteriosus
  - Ventricular septal defect and pulmonic stenosis
  - Transposition of the great vessels
  - Other causes of cyanosis with exercise intolerance

- ### Treatment
  - Endocarditis prophylaxis
  - Surgical correction
  - Rarely, palliative surgery (eg, Blalock-Taussig shunt; systemic artery to pulmonary artery)

- ### Pearl

Common associated anomalies include ASD (15%), right-sided aortic arch (25%), and anomalous coronary distribution (10%).

Reference

Maeda J et al: Frequent association of 22q11.2 deletion with tetralogy of Fallot. Am J Med Genet 2000;94:269.

Total Anomalous Pulmonary Venous Drainage

- **Essentials of Diagnosis**
  - Infant with cyanosis or congestive heart failure, depending on the size of the interatrial communication and whether the pulmonary venous channel is obstructed
  - Hyperdynamic right ventricular impulse with wide fixed split second heart sound and a third sound; systolic ejection murmur along the left sternal border and a diastolic flow rumble across the tricuspid valve
  - Right-heart chamber enlargement on ECG
  - Right-heart enlargement and pulmonary vascular engorgement on chest radiograph

- **Differential Diagnosis**
  - ASD
  - Pentalogy of Fallot (tetralogy plus ASD)
  - Other causes of cyanosis and heart failure

- **Treatment**
  - Balloon atrial septostomy and aggressive medical therapy for palliation
  - Definitive surgical repair

- **Pearl**

The confluence of pulmonary veins in total anomalous pulmonary venous drainage usually drains into 1 of 3 structures: the left innominate vein, the coronary sinus, or the portal vein. In most cases, it drains into the left innominate vein through a persistent left superior vena cava (vertical vein). The pulmonary venous confluence, the vertical vein, and the left innominate vein form a round shadow above the cardiac mass, giving a "snowman" shape to the cardiac silhouette on the anterior-posterior chest radiograph.

Reference

Bando K et al: Surgical management of total anomalous pulmonary venous connection: Thirty year trends. Circulation 1995;94(suppl II):12.

Transposition of the Great Arteries

- **Essentials of Diagnosis**
  - History of cyanosis that worsens shortly after birth at the time of ductal closure
  - Prominent right ventricular impulse, palpable and delayed A_2; murmurs from associated defects (eg, ventricular septal defect, pulmonic stenosis)
  - Chest radiograph shows narrowing at base of heart in region of great vessels; prominent pulmonary vascularity unless pulmonary vascular resistance is increased
  - Right atrial enlargement, right ventricular hypertrophy; occasionally biventricular hypertrophy (with an associated ventricular septal defect)
  - Great arteries are discordant, with anterior and rightward aorta arising from the right ventricle and leftward and posterior pulmonary artery arising from the left ventricle. Atria and ventricles are usually in normal position with severe right ventricular hypertrophy.

- **Differential Diagnosis**
  - Truncus arteriosus
  - Tetralogy of Fallot
  - Eisenmenger syndrome
  - Other causes of cyanosis

- **Treatment**
  - Surgical correction involves switching the great vessels (Jatene repair)
  - The atrial switch operations (Mustard, Senning) are less favored today because of the high incidence of late complications and the need for the anatomic right ventricle to supply the systemic circulation

- **Pearl**

About 20% of patients with transposition of the great arteries have anomalous coronary artery originations.

Reference

Losasy J et al: Late outcome after arterial switch operation for transposition of the great arteries. Circulation 2001;104:121I.

Tricuspid Atresia

- ■ Essentials of Diagnosis
  - • History of either cyanosis (70%) or congestive heart failure (30%)
  - • Cyanotic patient with absent right ventricular impulse and prominent left ventricular impulse
  - • Oligemic lung fields, right atrial and left ventricular prominence without right ventricular enlargement in retrosternal air space on chest radiograph
  - • Evidence of left ventricular hypertrophy, absent or atretic tricuspid valve, ASD, small right ventricle

- ■ Differential Diagnosis
  - • Ebstein anomaly with intermittent cyanosis
  - • Pulmonary atresia with intact ventricular septum
  - • Transposition of the great arteries
  - • Other causes of cyanosis and heart failure

- ■ Treatment
  - • Palliative surgery to increase pulmonary blood flow, such as the Fontan procedure (cavocaval baffle to pulmonary artery connection) or Glenn procedure (superior cavopulmonary anastomosis)

- ■ Pearl

About 30% of patients with tricuspid atresia also have transposition of the great vessels and a ventricular septal defect. They present as infants with congestive heart failure and need pulmonary artery banding to prevent irreversible pulmonary hypertension and allow repair of the defects later.

Reference

Mair DD et al: The Fontan procedure for tricuspid atresia: Early and late results of a 25-year experience with 216 patients. J Am Coll Cardiol 2001;37:933.

Truncus Arteriosus

- ■ Essentials of Diagnosis
  - Clinical presentation is congestive heart failure or cyanosis, depending on pulmonary blood flow and associated lesions
  - Imaging studies show a single great vessel arising from the heart and a single semilunar valve that gives rise to the aorta and the pulmonary and coronary arteries
  - Thirty percent of patients have DiGeorge syndrome and chromosome 22q11 deletion; truncal valve regurgitation occurs in half
  - In one third, the truncal valve is bicuspid or quadricuspid

- ■ Differential Diagnosis
  - Tetralogy of Fallot with pulmonary atresia (pseudotruncus)
  - Aortopulmonary septal defect or window
  - Origin of the right pulmonary artery from the aorta
  - Other causes of cyanosis or heart failure

- ■ Treatment
  - Surgical repair can be done early for infants with heart failure or severe truncal regurgitation
  - When conduits are used, they may need to be replaced with larger ones in 5–10 years

- ■ Pearl

DiGeorge syndrome consists of parathyroid hypoplasia, hypocalcemia, convulsions, peculiar faces (small mouth and chin, narrow eyes, and deformed ears), and cardiac abnormalities. These patients often have truncus arteriosis, peripheral pulmonary stenosis, absence of 1 pulmonary artery (Van Praagh type A3), and aortopulmonary collaterals.

Reference

Momma K et al: Truncus arteriosus communis associated with chromosome 22q11 deletion. J Am Coll Cardiol 1997;30:1067.

Ventricular Septal Defect

- ■ Essentials of Diagnosis
    - • History of murmur appearing shortly after birth
    - • Holosystolic murmur at left sternal border, radiating rightward
    - • Left atrial and left ventricular or biventricular enlargement
    - • High-velocity color-flow Doppler jet across ventricular septal defect
    - • Increased pulmonary flow velocities

- ■ Differential Diagnosis
    - • Other causes of exertional dyspnea
    - • Other causes of pulmonary hypertension
    - • Tricuspid regurgitation
    - • Mitral regurgitation

- ■ Treatment
    - • Antibiotic prophylaxis for infective endocarditis
    - • Surgical correction for left-to-right shunts greater than 2:1
    - • Pulmonary hypertension increases the risk of surgery

- ■ Pearl

A defect in the supracristal membranous septum can result in herniation of the right aortic sinus, leading to marked aortic regurgitation.

Reference

Neumayer U et al: Small ventricular septal defects in adults. Eur Heart J 1998;19:1573.

Arrhythmias

Atrial Fibrillation

- **Essentials of Diagnosis**
  - Irregularly irregular ventricular rhythm
  - Absence of P waves on the electrocardiogram (ECG)
  - The most common chronic arrhythmia
  - Common causes include hypertensive heart disease, systolic dysfunction of any cause, mitral valve disease, cardiac surgery, hyperthyroidism, and idiopathic (lone atrial fibrillation)
  - Variable S1, Occasional S3, and absent S4
  - Palpitations, chest pain, and shortness of breath

- **Differential Diagnosis**
  - Multifocal atrial tachycardia
  - Atrial flutter with variable atrioventricular (AV) block
  - Sinus rhythm with consecutive premature atrial contractions

- **Treatment**
  - Ventricular rate control with beta-blockers, calcium channel blockers, and digoxin either alone or in combination
  - Choice of therapy depends on left ventricular function (avoid class IC in patients with ischemic heart disease or ibutilide and class IC in patients with severe left ventricular dysfunction)
  - Acute intravenous (IV) esmolol or diltiazem for rate control
  - Cardioversion with countershock in unstable patients
  - Elective cardioversion with countershock or antiarrhythmic agents (IV ibutilide, procainamide, amiodarone; or oral propafenone 600 mg or flecainide 300 mg as single dose) once left atrial thrombus has been excluded by transesophageal echocardiography or patient has received adequate anticoagulation for 3–4 weeks
  - Anticoagulation for 4 weeks in postcardioversion patients
  - Chronic anticoagulation in all patients except lone atrial fibrillation (age <60 years and no structural heart disease) unless there is a serious contraindication (in which case give at least aspirin)
  - Rate control with anticoagulation is equivalent to rhythm control with antiarrhythmic agents regarding death and cardiovascular morbidity

- **Pearl**

Atrial fibrillation is uncommon in acute myocardial infarction and usually implies concomitant pericarditis.

Reference

Prystowsky EN: Management of atrial fibrillation: Therapeutic options and clinical decisions. Am J Cardiol 2000;85:3D.

Atrial Flutter

- ■ Essentials of Diagnosis
  - Regular ventricular rate of 75–150 beats per minute (bpm)
  - Irregular ventricular response secondary to variable AV block, usually induced by medication
  - Prominent neck vein pulsations of about 300/min
  - Flutter waves ("saw-tooth" in lead II) on ECG of 250–340/min

- ■ Differential Diagnosis
  - Atrial tachycardia
  - Paroxysmal supraventricular tachycardia

- ■ Treatment
  - Chronic anticoagulation with warfarin for stroke prevention
  - Restoration of sinus rhythm with electrical cardioversion or over-drive pacing
  - Chemical cardioversion with IV ibutilide
  - Flecainide 300 mg or propafenone 600 mg orally as single dose to restore sinus rhythm (used in patients with structurally normal hearts)
  - Rate control with beta-blockers, calcium channel blockers, or digoxin either individually or in combination
  - Radiofrequency ablation is curative in 90%

- ■ Pearl

In any regular narrow QRS tachycardia with a ventricular rate of about 150 bpm, atrial flutter must be in the differential diagnosis.

Reference

Cosio FG et al: Radiofrequency ablation of atrial flutter. J Cardiovasc Electrophysiol 1996;7:60.

Atrioventricular Nodal-His Block

- Essentials of Diagnosis
  - First degree: prolonged PR interval greater than 0.20 second
  - Second degree, Type I (Mobitz): progressive increase in P-R interval, then failure of AV conduction and absent QRS complex
  - Second degree, Type II (Mobitz): abrupt failure of AV conduction not preceded by increasing PR intervals
  - High degree: AV conduction ratio greater than 3:1
  - Complete or third degree: independent atrial and ventricular rhythms, with failure of AV conduction despite temporal opportunity for it to occur
  - Common causes: degenerative process, ischemia, calcific aortic valve disease, AV node ablative procedures, and medications
  - Symptoms of AV block: syncope, lightheadedness, and confusion
  - Clinical signs of complete AV block: cannon *a* waves in the jugular venous pulse and variable first heart sound intensity

- Differential Diagnosis & Causes
  - Causes of Mobitz I and first-degree AV block: increased vagal tone; drugs that prolong AV conduction such as beta-blockers, digoxin, and calcium channel blockers
  - Causes of Mobitz II and third-degree AV block: degenerative conduction system disease (Lev disease and Lenègre syndrome)
  - Acute myocardial infarction: inferior myocardial infarction causes complete heart block at the AV node; anterior myocardial infarction causes heart block distal to it
  - Other causes: acute myocarditis (viral, Lyme disease), digoxin toxicity, congenital

- Treatment
  - Pacemaker for symptoms of cerebral hypoperfusion
  - Pacemaker for symptomatic patients with Mobitz II and complete heart block
  - No treatment for most patients with Mobitz I block unless they progress or develop symptoms

- Pearl

A 2:1 AV block may be Mobitz I or II block. Prolonged QRS interval suggests that the block is infra-His in location, and, if symptomatic, a pacemaker is indicated.

Reference

Hayes DL: Evolving indications for permanent pacing. Am J Cardiol 1999;83:161D.

Atrioventricular Nodal Reentrant Tachycardia

- **Essentials of Diagnosis**
  - Heart rate 100–200 bpm or more
  - Neck pulsations corresponding to the heart rate
  - P waves not visible in 90% of cases
  - Occasionally, retrograde P waves are seen after the QRS complex or buried within the end of the QRS complex
  - Short RP tachycardia (RP interval shorter than PR interval)
  - In atypical AV nodal reentrant tachycardia (<10% of cases), long RP tachycardia (RP interval greater than PR interval) may be seen

- **Differential Diagnosis**
  - AV reentrant tachycardia
  - Atrial tachycardia

- **Treatment**
  - Acute termination occurs with adenosine 6-mg or 12-mg bolus injection
  - Maintenance therapy includes beta-blockers or calcium channel blockers to inhibit the slow pathway
  - Class I drugs may be used to inhibit the fast pathway
  - Radiofrequency ablation offers a cure rate of 95%

- **Pearl**

Adenosine is useful to treat a narrow QRS complex tachycardia, but even when it is ineffective, it might provide clues to the mechanism of tachycardia. If the tachycardia does not terminate after adenosine administration, the AV node is not part of the reentrant pathway.

Reference

Tebbenjohannas J et al: Noninvasive diagnosis in patients with undocumented tachycardias: Value of the adenosine test to predict AV nodal reentrant tachycardia. J Cardiovasc Electrophysiol 1999;10:916.

Atrioventricular Reciprocating Tachycardia: Bypass Tracts & Wolff-Parkinson-White Syndrome

- **Essentials of Diagnosis**
  - Short P-R interval (<120 ms)
  - Wide QRS complex caused by a delta wave
  - Supraventricular tachycardias with heart rates of 140–250 bpm
  - 5–10% have structural heart disease (Ebstein anomaly is the most common)
  - When the bypass tract conducts retrograde (antegrade conduction over the AV node), AV reciprocating tachycardia (AVRT) results
  - Orthodromic AVRT (antegrade over AV node) accounts for 70–80% and antidromic (retrograde over AV node) accounts for 5–10%
  - Orthodromic tachycardia has a narrow QRS complex, and antidromic tachycardia has a wide QRS complex
  - Multiple accessory pathways are associated with a higher incidence of ventricular fibrillation
  - Atrial fibrillation with accessory pathway is potentially lethal
  - Minimum R-R interval less than 250 ms during atrial fibrillation is a marker of sudden death
  - Concealed bypass tracts conduct retrograde only and cause orthodromic AVRT, but cannot be detected during sinus rhythm

- **Differential Diagnosis**
  - AV nodal reentrant tachycardia
  - Supraventricular tachycardia with aberrancy

- **Treatment**
  - For regular narrow QRS tachycardia, adenosine 6–12 mg is useful to terminate the arrhythmia
  - Drugs that block the AV node, when used independently, may facilitate the conduction of atrial fibrillation through the accessory pathway, resulting in ventricular fibrillation
  - Recurrent regular narrow QRS tachycardia may be treated with beta-blockers or calcium channel blockers
  - Digoxin must be avoided because it may improve conduction over the accessory pathway
  - Class IA, class IC, or amiodarone may be tried to control arrhythmia with antidromic mechanism
  - For recurrent arrhythmia, radiofrequency ablation has a high success rate (95%)

- **Pearl**

For atrial fibrillation in a young patient, IV procainamide or ibutilide should be used preferentially.

Reference

Al-Khatib SM, Pritchett EL: Clinical features of Wolff-Parkinson-White syndrome. Am Heart J 1999;138:403.

Automatic (Ectopic) Atrial Tachycardia

- **Essentials of Diagnosis**
  - Heart rate 100–180 bpm
  - P waves different from sinus P waves
  - Initiated by ectopic beat
  - Gradual increase in heart rate during an episode
  - Continuous tachycardia may cause tachycardia cardiomyopathy, mostly in children

- **Differential Diagnosis**
  - Reentrant atrial tachycardia
  - Atypical AV nodal reentrant tachycardia

- **Treatment**
  - Sotalol is the best choice, followed by flecainide
  - Propafenone and amiodarone are alternative choices
  - Beta-blockers are effective to slow the ventricular rate
  - Verapamil and digoxin are uniformly ineffective
  - Radiofrequency ablation is effective

- **Pearl**

For a young patient with cardiomyopathy, consider automatic atrial tachycardia in the differential diagnosis.

Reference

Marchlinski F et al: Magnetic electroanatomical mapping for ablation of focal atrial tachycardias. Pacing Clin Electrophysiol 1998;21:1621.

Brugada Syndrome

- **Essentials of Diagnosis**
  - Life-threatening cardiac arrhythmia (ventricular fibrillation and ventricular tachycardia) with no demonstrable structural cardiac disease
  - Apparent right bundle branch block with ST elevation in V1–V3 (V2 always present)
  - The disease is secondary to a mutation in the sodium channel (*SCN5A*)
  - Flecainide or procainamide may be used to unmask the ECG changes (ST elevation in V2)

- **Differential Diagnosis**
  - Long QT syndrome
  - Idiopathic ventricular arrhythmia
  - The ECG changes may mimic acute myocardial infarction (cardiac enzymes and regional wall motion are usually normal, but may be transiently abnormal after a cardiac arrest)

- **Treatment**
  - Implantable cardioverter-defibrillator is needed for patients with life-threatening arrhythmia
  - Asymptomatic patients with abnormal ECG at baseline require electrophysiologic studies; if sustained ventricular arrhythmia is inducible, an implantable cardioverter-defibrillator is recommended
  - Asymptomatic patients with normal baseline ECG require no further testing

- **Pearl**

Not all ST elevations indicate myocardial injury. Although the disease is uncommon, think of Brugada syndrome in the appropriate setting (young patient with cardiac arrest, abnormal ECG, and structurally normal heart).

Reference

Wilde AA et al: Proposed diagnostic criteria for the Brugada syndrome. Eur Heart J 2002;23:1648.

Bundle Branch Reentrant Ventricular Tachycardia

- **Essentials of Diagnosis**
  - Rapid ventricular tachycardia, usually with left bundle branch block morphology
  - The impulse reenters within the conduction system
  - 90% right bundle antegrade and left bundle retrograde conduction
  - 10% left bundle antegrade and right bundle retrograde conduction
  - Generally occurs with advanced nonischemic dilated cardiomyopathy
  - The arrhythmia usually causes symptoms; patients often present with syncope or cardiac arrest
  - Intraventricular conduction system disease is common
  - HV interval during the tachycardia is usually the same as in sinus rhythm

- **Differential Diagnosis**
  - Intramyocardial reentrant ventricular tachycardia
  - Supraventricular tachycardia with aberrancy
  - Mahaim tachycardia

- **Treatment**
  - Right bundle branch ablation
  - Cardioverter-defibrillator is implanted concurrent with ablation because of the risk for sudden death with poor left ventricular function

- **Pearl**

Bundle branch reentry should be suspected as a cause of ventricular tachycardia in a patient with nonischemic dilated cardiomyopathy.

Reference

Tchou P, Mehdirad AA: Bundle branch reentry ventricular tachycardia. Pacing Clin Electrophysiol 1995;18:1427.

Carotid Sinus Hypersensitivity

■ Essentials of Diagnosis

- Syncope tends to be abrupt, and patient may not recall a specific maneuver
- Occurs in older patients
- Bradycardia and vasodepressor element may both play a role
- Precipitating events such as shaving or looking up may be reported
- Carotid aneurysm and head-neck tumors can predispose
- May present as unexplained falls
- Frequently associated with coronary artery disease

■ Differential Diagnosis

- Neurocardiogenic syncope
- Ventricular tachycardia may coexist with carotid sinus hypersensitivity, particularly in patients with previous myocardial infarction or systolic dysfunction

■ Treatment

- Elimination of triggers such as tight collars
- Avoidance of diuretics and negative chronotropic drugs when feasible
- Pacemaker
- Adjuvant treatment with serotonin reuptake inhibitors in patients with a substantial vasodepressor element

■ Pearl

In an elderly patient with unexplained falls, consider this diagnosis and perform carotid sinus massage with ECG monitoring.

Reference

Fahmy RN et al: Revisiting carotid sinus denervation in carotid sinus hypersensitivity. Am Heart J 1995;130:1318.

Effort Syncope

- ■ Essentials of Diagnosis
  - Sudden transient loss of consciousness during exercise, especially unaccustomed exercise, with rapid spontaneous recovery
  - Absence of prodromal symptoms
  - History of heart disease, heart murmurs, or other cardiac symptoms

- ■ Differential Diagnosis & Causes
  - Severe aortic stenosis
  - Hypertrophic obstructive cardiomyopathy
  - Discrete subaortic stenosis or supravalvular aortic stenosis
  - Severe mitral stenosis
  - Severe pulmonic stenosis
  - Severe pulmonary hypertension
  - Intracardiac tumors
  - Arrhythmia-induced syncope
  - Transient myocardial ischemia
  - Severe left ventricular dysfunction

- ■ Treatment
  - Treat the underlying condition
  - Avoid unaccustomed exertion

- ■ Pearl

A spontaneously provided history of effort syncope is unusual because many patients experience it only once. Whatever patients were doing at the time, they never do it again.

Reference

Haner KE: Discovering the cause of syncope. A guide to the focused evaluation. Postgrad Med 2003;113:31.

Implanted Cardioverter-Defibrillator, Frequent Discharges

- ## Essentials of Diagnosis
  - Appropriate therapy for recurrent ventricular arrhythmia
  - Supraventricular arrhythmia including sinus tachycardia and atrial fibrillation with rapid ventricular response
  - Frequent and inappropriate discharges of implanted cardioverter-defibrillator

- ## Differential Diagnosis & Causes
  Cardiac causes
  - T-wave or P-wave oversensing
  - Double counting of intrinsic wide QRS complex in biventricular defibrillator

  Noncardiac causes
  - Myopotential oversensing (eg, diaphragm)
  - Device–device interaction (sensing of pacemaker stimuli)
  - Device malfunction
  - Electromagnetic interference

- ## Treatment
  - If appropriate, consider altering the substrate with antiarrhythmic drugs or ablation
  - Exclude or treat precipitating factors such as metabolic derangement, ischemia, and thyroid dysfunction
  - If the cause is rhythm misinterpretation or device malfunction, manage appropriately with electrophysiology consultation

- ## Pearl
  If a patient is frequently shocked inappropriately in the hospital, place a magnet over the device to eliminate the sensing function and thereby stop further shocks until definitive treatment.

Reference

Gollob MH, Seger JJ: Current status of the implantable cardioverter-defibrillator. Chest 2001;119:1210.

Intra-atrial Reentrant Tachycardia

- **Essentials of Diagnosis**
  - Atrial rate of 120–240 bpm
  - P waves different from sinus P wave
  - Most patients have structural heart disease

- **Differential Diagnosis**
  - Automatic atrial tachycardia
  - Atypical AV nodal reentrant tachycardia

- **Treatment**
  - Beta-blockers or calcium channel blockers with negative chronotropic properties (verapamil or diltiazem)
  - Amiodarone, class IC, class IA, and other class III drugs are alternates when this arrhythmia is difficult to control
  - Radiofrequency ablation
  - In difficult circumstances, AV node ablation with implantation of a pacemaker

- **Pearl**

Reentrant atrial tachycardia following cardiac surgery (incisional tachycardia) is increasing in incidence.

Reference

Haines DE, DiMarco JP: Sustained intraatrial reentrant tachycardia: Clinical, electrocardiographic, and electrophysiologic characteristics and long-term follow-up. J Am Coll Cardiol 1990;15:1345.

Long QT Syndrome

- Essentials of Diagnosis
  - Clinical constellation of congenital deafness, prolongation of the QT interval ($QT_c > 480$ ms), syncope, and sudden death
  - Family history of sudden death
  - Characteristic arrhythmia is torsades de pointes
  - The fundamental abnormality is prolongation of action potential secondary to abnormality of transmembrane ion transport
  - Emotion seems to trigger cardiac events, particularly in patients with *KvLQT1*

- Differential Diagnosis
  - Metabolic abnormalities with prolongation of QT
  - Drug-induced long QT
  - Idiopathic ventricular arrhythmia

- Treatment
  - Beta-blockers
  - Sympathetic denervation
  - Adjuvant pacemaker therapy
  - Implantation of cardioverter-defibrillator in those with syncope or cardiac arrest during adrenergic modulation (beta-blockers and sympathectomy), or when the first event is a documented cardiac arrest

- Pearl

In young patients with syncope, exclude long QT interval as a cause with ECG and a careful family history.

Reference

Passman R et al: Polymorphic ventricular tachycardia, long Q-T syndrome, and torsades de pointes. Med Clin North Am 2001;85:321.

Multifocal Atrial Tachycardia

- ### Essentials of Diagnosis
  - Heart rates up to 150 bpm
  - Three or more distinct P waves in a single lead
  - Variable P-P, P-R, and R-R intervals
  - 60–85% of cases are associated with pulmonary disease

- ### Differential Diagnosis
  - Atrial fibrillation

- ### Treatment
  - Treat the underlying cause (ie, respiratory failure)
  - Verapamil is useful
  - Beta-blockers may be used for ventricular rate control if tolerated

- ### Pearl

In patients with chronic lung disease, carefully differentiate multifocal atrial tachycardia from atrial fibrillation; the latter requires anticoagulation but the former does not.

Reference

Tucker KJ et al: Treatment of refractory recurrent multifocal atrial tachycardia with atrioventricular junction ablation and permanent pacing. J Invasive Cardiol 1995;7:207.

Neurocardiogenic Syncope

- **Essentials of Diagnosis**
  - Most common mechanism of syncope in the young
  - Bradycardia (vagal) and profound hypotension (vasodepressor) may occur either alone or in varying proportions
  - Pain, fear, or emotion may precipitate syncope
  - Many spells over several years are suggestive of this disorder
  - Tilt testing is useful in the diagnosis

- **Differential diagnosis**
  - Sick sinus syndrome
  - Orthostatic hypotension
  - Iatrogenic syncope caused by antihypertensive medications

- **Treatment**
  - Salt and fluid loading; avoidance of dehydration
  - Fludrocortisone
  - Beta-blockers
  - Adrenergic agonist midodrine
  - Serotonin reuptake inhibitors
  - Disopyramide
  - Pacemaker

- **Pearl**

Recurrent syncope with no sequelae and onset at a young age are suggestive of neurocardiogenic syncope.

Reference

Goldschlager N et al: Etiologic considerations in the patient with syncope and an apparently normal heart. Arch Intern Med 2003;163:151.

Nonparoxysmal Junctional Tachycardia (Accelerated Atrioventricular Junctional Rhythm)

- **Essentials of Diagnosis**
  - Heart rate 60–120 bpm
  - AV dissociation
  - Gradual onset and termination
  - When rhythm is caused by digoxin, AV dissociation is common
  - Usually seen with organic heart disease
  - Causes include digoxin, inferior myocardial infarction, open-heart surgery, myocarditis, and rarely congenital heart disease

- **Differential Diagnosis**
  - Atrial tachycardia

- **Treatment**
  - No treatment is usually indicated
  - Rhythm spontaneously resolves as the inciting event subsides
  - If the rhythm is hemodynamically disturbing, AV sequential pacing at a rate faster than the tachycardia may suppress the rhythm and restore the atrial contribution to cardiac output

- **Pearl**

Therapeutic nihilism is not a bad choice in some arrhythmias.

Reference

Ruder MA et al: Clinical and electrophysiologic characterization of automatic junctional tachycardia in adults. Circulation 1986;73:930.

Orthostatic Hypotension

- ■ Essentials of Diagnosis
  - • Symptoms of reduced cerebral perfusion upon assuming an upright position: dizziness to frank syncope
  - • Marked fall in blood pressure upon standing (>20 mm Hg systolic or >10 mm Hg diastolic)

- ■ Differential Diagnosis & Causes
  - • Fluid loss, anemia, dehydration
  - • Primary autonomic dysfunction: Shy-Drager syndrome
  - • Secondary dysautonomia: Parkinson disease, diabetes mellitus, amyloidosis, human immunodeficiency virus infection, multiple sclerosis
  - • Vasoactive medications: antihypertensive agents, ethanol, psychoactive drugs
  - • Advanced age: akinetic falling spells of the aged

- ■ Treatment
  - • Treat underlying cause if possible
  - • Wear elastic stockings
  - • Maintain adequate salt and water intake
  - • Administer fludrocortisone
  - • Give alpha-1-adrenergic agonists

- ■ Pearl

Always measure orthostatic blood pressure changes (remember the maximum effect is between 90 and 180 seconds) in patients with dizziness or syncope. This can save the patient the inconvenience and expense of an extensive evaluation.

Reference

Pavri BB, Ho RT: Syncope. Identifying cardiac causes in older patients. Geriatrics 2003;58:26.

Other Bypass Tracts: Atriofascicular Tachycardia (Mahaim Tachycardia)

- **Essentials of Diagnosis**
  - Wide QRS tachycardia (left bundle branch block and superior-axis morphology)
  - Diagnosis confirmed at electrophysiologic study
  - Progressive decrease in AV conduction (anterograde decremental conduction)
  - Coexistence with AV nodal reentrant tachycardia and other accessory pathways

- **Differential Diagnosis**
  - Ventricular tachycardia

- **Treatment**
  - Radiofrequency ablation

- **Pearl**

Termination of tachycardia by adenosine administration does not exclude ventricular tachycardia.

Reference

Aliot E et al: Mahaim tachycardias. Eur Heart J 1998;19:E25.

Pacemaker Malfunction

- **Essentials of Diagnosis**
  - Failure to capture: pacing spike is not followed by a depolarization
  - Oversensing: typically the T wave or skeletal muscle potentials are sensed as depolarization, and a pacing spike is not initiated
  - Pacemaker-mediated tachycardia: Pacing at or near the programmed upper rate limit secondary to retrograde conduction of the ventricular complex to the atrium, which is sensed as a P wave
  - Lead fracture is suspected when there is high impedance
  - Lead insulation failure leads to low lead impedance
  - Electromagnetic interference (eg, by antitheft devices) may interfere with pacemaker function

- **Differential Diagnosis**
  - Lead dislodgment
  - Loose connection between the lead and pulse generator
  - Metabolic abnormalities such as hyperkalemia
  - Antiarrhythmic medication

- **Treatment**
  - Treatment depends on the cause of malfunction
  - Pacemaker-mediated tachycardia can be treated by prolongation of the postventricular atrial refractory period

- **Pearl**

Patients with pacemakers should not linger around anti-theft devices in stores.

Reference

Hayes DL, Vlietstra RE: Pacemaker malfunction. Ann Intern Med 1993;119:828.

Pacemaker Syndrome

- **Essentials of Diagnosis**
  - Weakness, orthopnea, dizziness, breathlessness, presyncope, syncope, pulmonary congestion, and altered mental status
  - Atrial rhythm and rate are dyssynchronous with the ventricular rhythm and rate
  - Appropriately timed atrial contraction does not precede the paced ventricular event
  - Prevalence is 10–50% and more common in the elderly
  - Common with VVI pacing and reduced with dual-chamber pacing
  - Diagnosis established by the objective findings of ventricular-atrial conduction, cannon waves, and transient mitral regurgitation
  - Ambulatory monitoring may be useful in confirming the diagnosis
  - Atrial contraction and resultant atrial stretch activate the baroreceptors to produce vagally mediated vasodilation and decrease in heart rate

- **Differential Diagnosis**
  - Newer forms of pacemaker syndromes such as prolonged AV conduction (intrinsic AV node problem or drug induced) in AAI or AAIR mode
  - AV dyssynchrony caused by mode switching

- **Treatment**
  - Atrial pacing and sensing unless contraindicated
  - In VVI pacing, upgrading to DDD mode with physiologic AV pace intervals
  - Reducing the lower rate of VVI pacing to reduce the number of paced events
  - Trial of antiarrhythmic drugs to eliminate retrograde ventriculoatrial conduction

- **Pearl**

For elderly patients with episodes of altered mental status and a pacemaker, consider this syndrome in the differential diagnosis.

Reference

Mitrani RD et al: Cardiac pacemakers: Current and future status. Curr Probl Cardiol 1999;24:341.

Paroxysmal Atrial Tachycardia with Block

- ■ Essentials of Diagnosis
  - • Atrial rate of 150–250 bpm
  - • AV block of 2:1
  - • Often associated with digitalis toxicity

- ■ Differential Diagnosis
  - • Other forms of atrial tachycardia
  - • Atypical AV nodal reentrant tachycardia
  - • Atrial flutter

- ■ Treatment
  - • Withdraw digoxin when appropriate
  - • Correct electrolyte abnormalities
  - • Therapies targeted at abolishing the arrhythmia are unrewarding

- ■ Pearl

This is the most commonly missed rhythm disturbance because the ventricular rate is often in the normal range as a result of AV block and the second P wave is overlooked.

Reference

Spodick DH: Electrocardiology teacher analysis and review: Atrial flutter vs. (paroxysmal) atrial tachycardia with block. Am J Geriatr Cardiol 1999;8:143.

Permanent Form of Junctional Reciprocating Tachycardia

- **Essentials of Diagnosis**
  - Commonly observed in children
  - Heart rate may vary from 120 to 250 bpm
  - Tachycardia cardiomyopathy may occur because the tachycardia tends to be incessant
  - This is a reentrant tachycardia and quite sensitive to autonomic manipulation
  - Tachycardia tends to slow down with age because retrograde conduction through the accessory pathway tends to slow down

- **Differential Diagnosis**
  - Automatic atrial tachycardia
  - Atypical AV nodal reentrant tachycardia

- **Treatment**
  - Drug therapy is frequently unhelpful
  - Type 1C drug or amiodarone may achieve rate control
  - Digoxin has no effect, and verapamil may accelerate the tachycardia
  - Beta-blockers may control heart rate in adults
  - Radiofrequency ablation is successful in 95% of patients

- **Pearl**

Consider this arrhythmia in a young adult with cardiomyopathy.

Reference

Critelli G: Recognizing and managing permanent junctional reciprocating tachycardia in the catheter ablation era. J Cardiovasc Electrophysiol 1997;8:226.

Postural Tachycardia Syndrome

- **Essentials of Diagnosis**
  - Chronic orthostatic symptoms with a dramatic rise in heart rate (>30 bpm) on standing, with absence of orthostatic hypotension; frank syncope is rare
  - Evidence of dysautonomia on functional testing

- **Differential Diagnosis**
  - Orthostatic hypotension
  - Neurocardiogenic syndrome
  - Chronic fatigue syndrome
  - Other neuropathies (eg, syringomyelia)
  - Supraventricular tachyarrhythmias

- **Treatment**
  - Salt and fluid replacement
  - Fludrocortisone
  - Autonomic agents: alpha-1-adrenergic agonists, cardioselective beta-blockers

- **Pearl**

Full recovery is possible, especially if an antecedent viral infection is identified.

Reference

Jacob G et al: The neuropathic postural tachycardia syndrome. N Engl J Med 2000;343:1008.

Sinus Arrhythmia

- **Essentials of Diagnosis**
  - Cyclic heart rate variation with respiration
  - Nonrespiratory form may be related to sick sinus syndrome or digitalis intoxication
  - Variability of P-P cycle length at least 160 ms or 10% of the minimum cycle length
  - P-wave morphology identical to normal sinus rhythm
  - Seen in young patients or those treated with digitalis or morphine
  - Rarely associated with increased intracranial pressure

- **Differential Diagnosis**
  - Sinoatrial exit block
  - Sinus pause

- **Treatment**
  - Treat the underlying cause
  - Withdraw the offending drug

- **Pearl**

Ventriculophasic sinus arrhythmia is a unique form of sinus arrhythmia. This is diagnosed when P-P intervals containing a QRS complex are shorter than those that do not. It usually occurs when the ventricular rate is slow and independent. It does not cause serious hemodynamic changes.

Reference

Chakko S, Kessler KM: Recognition and management of cardiac arrhythmias. Curr Probl Cardiol 1995;20:53.

Sinus Bradycardia

- ■ Essentials of Diagnosis
  - Sinus rate is less than 60 bpm
  - P waves have normal contour with a constant PR interval
  - PR interval exceeds 120 ms
  - Sinus arrhythmia often coexists
  - High vagal tone (young adults and athletes) or medications (eg, beta-blockers) may cause sinus bradycardia
  - Increased intracranial pressure and myxedema are among several other causes
  - Acute myocardial infarction (particularly inferior) is associated with sinus bradycardia

- ■ Differential Diagnosis
  - Ectopic atrial bradycardia

- ■ Treatment
  - Usually no specific treatment is needed
  - If patients are symptomatic acutely, atropine may be used to increase the sinus rate
  - Patients with recurrent symptoms are treated with a pacemaker

- ■ Pearl

Do not forget to exclude myxedema in symptomatic patients with sinus bradycardia.

Reference

Mangrum JM, DiMarco JP: The evaluation and management of bradycardia. N Engl J Med 2000;342:703.

Sinus Node Dysfunction

- **Essentials of Diagnosis**
  - Sinus bradycardia with rate less than 50 bpm
  - Sinoatrial exit block type I: progressively shorter P-P intervals, followed by failure of occurrence of a P wave
  - Sinoatrial exit block type II: pauses in sinus rhythm that are multiples of basic sinus rate
  - Sinus arrest or pause: failure of occurrence of P waves at expected times
  - Usually caused by a degenerative process associated with aging
  - Negative chronotropic drugs may cause a similar problem
  - Tachycardia-bradycardia syndrome (bradycardia secondary to sinus node dysfunction coupled with supraventricular arrhythmia such as atrial fibrillation)

- **Differential Diagnosis**
  - Blocked premature atrial contraction may resemble sinoatrial exit block
  - Marked sinus arrhythmia
  - Conditions with high vagal tone (eg, young athletic individual, cough, micturition)

- **Treatment**
  - Avoid or eliminate negative chronotropic drugs
  - Symptomatic patients without reversible cause will need a pacemaker
  - Although atrial pacing may be sufficient because most patients subsequently develop AV nodal disease, dual-chamber pacemakers are recommended

- **Pearl**

Asymptomatic sinus node dysfunction, regardless of the duration of the pause, may be followed clinically. The onset of symptoms indicates the need for a pacemaker.

Reference

Andersen HR et al: Long-term follow up of patients from a randomized trial of atrial versus ventricular pacing for sick sinus syndrome. Lancet 1997;350:1210.

Sinus Node Reentry

- ■ Essentials of Diagnosis
  - • Heart rate 100–160 bpm
  - • Each QRS is preceded by a P wave identical to the P wave of normal sinus rhythm
  - • Abrupt onset and termination
  - • Organic heart disease in many patients

- ■ Differential Diagnosis
  - • Sinus tachycardia
  - • Inappropriate sinus tachycardia
  - • Atrial tachycardia

- ■ Treatment
  - • Digoxin and calcium channel blockers are the most useful drugs
  - • Beta-blockers
  - • Radiofrequency ablation

- ■ Pearl

Abrupt onset and termination (reentrant arrhythmia) is a clue to the diagnosis.

Reference

Sanders WE Jr et al: Catheter ablation of sinoatrial node reentrant tachycardia. J Am Coll Cardiol 1994;23:926.

Sinus Tachycardia

- **Essentials of Diagnosis**
  - Heart rate 100–160 bpm
  - Each QRS is preceded by a P wave identical to the P wave of normal sinus rhythm
  - Physiologic response to exercise or adrenergic response to disease
  - Common causes are blood loss, volume depletion, hyperthyroidism, fever, sepsis, and hypotension

- **Differential Diagnosis**
  - Sinus node reentry
  - Atrial tachycardia

- **Treatment**
  - Treat the underlying cause

- **Pearl**

In women of child-bearing age, pregnancy must be in the differential diagnosis.

Reference

Cossu SF, Steinberg JS: Supraventricular tachyarrhythmias involving the sinus node: Clinical and electrophysiologic characteristics. Prog Cardiovasc Dis 1998;41:51.

Sinus Tachycardia, Inappropriate

- ■ Essentials of Diagnosis
  - Heart rates greater than 100 bpm at rest or with minimal exertion
  - P waves identical or nearly identical to sinus P wave
  - Chronic duration of symptoms
  - Exclusion of other causes of sinus tachycardia
  - Frequently seen in young female health care workers
  - May occur transiently after ablation of other supraventricular arrhythmias

- ■ Differential Diagnosis
  - Appropriate sinus tachycardia
  - Sinus node reentry
  - Atrial tachycardia

- ■ Treatment
  - High doses of beta-blockers (atenolol 100–200 mg/d)
  - Calcium channel blockers
  - Radiofrequency modification of sinoatrial node (high recurrence rate of 20–30%)
  - Complications of radiofrequency ablation include the need for a pacemaker and superior vena cava syndrome

- ■ Pearl

Exclude other causes before diagnosing inappropriate sinus tachycardia.

Reference

Sergio FC, Steinberg JS: Supraventricular tachyarrhythmias involving the sinus node: Clinical and electrophysiologic characteristics. Prog Cardiovasc Dis 1998;41:51.

Sudden Cardiac Death

- **Essentials of Diagnosis**
  - Unexpected death within an hour of onset of symptoms; if a patient is successfully resuscitated, then it is called a sudden-death episode
  - Primary electrical mechanisms include ventricular fibrillation, ventricular tachycardia, asystole, and pulseless electrical activity
  - Associated diseases include coronary artery disease, dilated cardiomyopathy, hypertrophic cardiomyopathy, arrhythmogenic right ventricular dysplasia, and primary electrophysiologic disorders such as long QT syndrome, Brugada syndrome, and idiopathic ventricular arrhythmia
  - May also be due to massive pulmonary embolism, rupture of an aortic aneurysm, or massive stroke
  - Once the patient is resuscitated, investigations should include noninvasive tests such as ECG and echocardiography. Further risk stratification may include coronary arteriography and invasive electrophysiologic studies.
  - Patients with ischemic heart disease at risk for sudden cardiac death may need investigations such as signal-averaged ECG, micro–T-wave alternans, heart rate variability, and Holter monitoring

- **Differential Diagnosis**
  - Syncope
  - In young patients, consider coronary artery anomalies, with intermittent ischemia giving rise to ventricular arrhythmia
  - Drug-induced torsades de pointes

- **Treatment**
  - Revascularization in appropriate patients
  - Implantable cardioverter-defibrillator in patients with cardiac disease because recurrence rates are high
  - Antiarrhythmic drugs as a group are not effective, but beta-blockers and amiodarone may play a role

- **Pearl**

Remember that erythromycin and antihistamines together may induce torsades de pointes.

Reference

Huikuri HV et al: Sudden death due to cardiac arrhythmias. N Engl J Med 2001;345:1473.

Syncope

- ■ Essentials of Diagnosis
  - • Sudden, unexpected, and transient loss of consciousness and postural tone
  - • Spontaneous and full recovery
  - • Important causes include valvular stenosis, hypertrophic cardiomyopathy, pulmonary emboli, bradyarrhythmias such as complete heart block, tachyarrhythmias such as ventricular tachycardia, neurocardiogenic syncope, and situational syncope such as cough or micturition syncope
  - • Iatrogenic causes include medications with negative chronotropic activity such as beta-blockers, orthostatic hypotension secondary to vasodilators, or pacemaker malfunction
  - • Investigations for identifying the cause should be guided by clinical history and examination
  - • Useful investigations include ECG, echocardiography, ambulatory ECG monitoring, ECG event recorder, implantable ECG loop recorder, head-up tilt testing, and electrophysiologic studies

- ■ Differential Diagnosis
  - • Seizures
  - • Glossopharyngeal neuralgia
  - • Metabolic states such as hypoglycemia
  - • Cerebrovascular disease such as vertebrobasilar insufficiency
  - • Psychiatric disorder with hyperventilation
  - • Akinetic falling spells of the aged

- ■ Treatment
  - • Treatment depends on the cause
  - • If possible, withdraw the offending agent
  - • Implant pacemaker for bradyarrhythmia and use radiofrequency ablation or implantable cardioverter-defibrillator for tachyarrhythmia
  - • Treat neurocardiogenic syncope with beta-blockers, volume expansion, vasoconstrictors such as midodrine, and a selective serotonin reuptake inhibitor such as sertraline (patient response may vary; tilt-table test may assist with treatment choice)

- ■ Pearl

Patients without an identifiable cause of syncope after extensive investigation have a good prognosis.

Reference

Kapoor WN: Current evaluation and management of syncope. Circulation 2002;106:1606.

Torsades de Pointes

- **Essentials of Diagnosis**
  - Pause-dependent polymorphic ventricular arrhythmia occurs in the presence of a prolonged QT interval (ECG pattern often resembles twisting around a point, hence the name)
  - Lightheadedness, syncope, and sudden death may occur
  - Lengthening of the pause-dependent action potential provides the substrate for the arrhythmia
  - QT prolongation may be induced by medications such as class IA and III antiarrhythmic drugs, antibiotics such as erythromycin, the phenothiazine group of drugs, and metabolic states such as hypokalemia and hypomagnesemia

- **Differential Diagnosis**
  - Polymorphic ventricular tachycardia secondary to acute ischemia (QT interval may be normal)
  - Catecholamine-dependent polymorphic ventricular arrhythmia

- **Treatment**
  - Patients with hemodynamic collapse require emergent electrical countershock
  - Stable patients can start with IV magnesium
  - For frequent pauses, consider temporary pacing or IV isoproterenol
  - Eliminate medications that prolong the QT interval

- **Pearl**

Many common drugs, particularly when used in combination (eg, erythromycin and antihistamines), may cause QT prolongation and precipitate torsades de pointes.

Reference

Walker BD et al: Congenital and acquired long QT syndromes. Can J Cardiol 2003;19:76.

Ventricular Arrhythmia, Idiopathic

- **Essentials of Diagnosis**
  - Ventricular tachycardia occurs with no evidence of structural heart disease on echocardiography
  - Tachycardia may be caused by triggered activity (right ventricular outflow tract tachycardia) or reentry (left ventricular tachycardia)
  - Triggered outflow tract tachycardias are dependent on cyclic adenosine monophosphate and respond to IV adenosine
  - Magnetic resonance imaging may be abnormal
  - Overall, the arrhythmia carries a benign prognosis
  - The most common is right ventricular outflow tract tachycardia and is recognized as a left bundle branch block pattern of ventricular tachycardia with inferior axis

- **Differential Diagnosis**
  - Intramyocardial reentrant ventricular tachycardia
  - Arrhythmogenic dysplasia
  - Mahaim tachycardia
  - Tachycardia following repair of tetralogy of Fallot

- **Treatment**
  - Beta-blockers or verapamil
  - Class IA, IC, or III antiarrhythmic agents
  - Radiofrequency ablation

- **Pearl**

Sensitivity to adenosine does not exclude ventricular tachycardia. Right ventricular outflow tract tachycardia is typically sensitive to adenosine.

Reference

Wall TS, Freedman RA: Ventricular tachycardia in structurally normal hearts. Curr Cardiol Rep 2002;4:388.

Ventricular Tachycardia

- **Essentials of Diagnosis**
  - Monomorphic ventricular tachycardia
  - Nonsustained: 3 or more consecutive QRS complexes of uniform configuration and of ventricular origin at a rate of more than 100 bpm
  - Sustained: lasts more than 30 seconds or requires intervention for termination
  - Polymorphic ventricular tachycardia: beat-to-beat variation in QRS configuration
  - Clinical manifestations include sudden cardiac death, syncope, and near syncope
  - Most common with ischemic substrate and depressed left ventricular function; idiopathic dilated cardiomyopathy is also a frequent cause
  - Bundle branch reentry occurs most often with idiopathic dilated cardiomyopathy
  - Ventricular tachycardia with a structurally normal heart is rare

- **Differential Diagnosis**
  - Supraventricular tachycardia with aberrancy
  - AV dissociation, presence of fusion beats, and duration of R wave to nadir of S wave greater than 65 ms (left bundle branch block type) and greater than 100 ms (right bundle branch block type) in chest leads help to differentiate ventricular tachycardia from supraventricular tachycardia with aberrancy
  - Wolff-Parkinson-White syndrome with antidromic tachycardia

- **Treatment**
  - Stable patients can receive IV amiodarone or lidocaine
  - Unstable patients (hypotension, congestive heart failure, or chest pain) need immediate synchronized cardioversion
  - For recurrent sustained ventricular tachycardia and survivors of sudden death, implantable cardioverter-defibrillator is indicated; amiodarone may be needed to reduce frequency of shocks
  - For recurrent nonsustained ventricular tachycardia or ischemic left ventricular dysfunction, consider electrophysiologic studies or implantable cardioverter-defibrillator for primary prevention

- **Pearl**

The initial beats of ventricular tachycardia may be slightly irregular. In patients with left ventricular dysfunction or a history of myocardial infarction, think twice before diagnosing supraventricular tachycardia with aberrancy; it is more likely ventricular tachycardia.

Reference

Saliba WI, Natale A: Ventricular tachycardia syndromes. Med Clin North Am 2001;85:267.

Wandering Atrial Pacemaker

- **Essentials of Diagnosis**
  - Progressive cyclic variation in P-wave morphology
  - Heart rate 60–100 bpm
  - Variation of P-wave morphology, P-P interval, and the P-R interval

- **Differential Diagnosis**
  - Multifocal atrial tachycardia (heart rate >100 bpm)

- **Treatment**
  - No specific treatment
  - Monitor and treat the underlying cause, such as sick sinus syndrome or lung disease

- **Pearl**

Young patients with high vagal tone may have this benign rhythm.

Reference

Sergio FC, Steinberg JS: Supraventricular tachyarrhythmias involving the sinus node: Clinical and electrophysiologic characteristics. Prog Cardiovasc Dis 1998;41:51.

Endocrine Diseases & the Heart

Acromegaly & the Heart

- **Essentials of Diagnosis**
  - Elevated somatomedin C
  - Inability to suppress growth hormone to less than 2 ng/mL during glucose tolerance test
  - Pituitary adenoma found on magnetic resonance imaging
  - Biventricular hypertrophy with systolic and diastolic dysfunction
  - Hypertension, diabetes, and premature coronary artery disease

- **Differential Diagnosis**
  - Other causes of cardiomyopathy and heart failure
  - Other causes of hypertension
  - Other causes of premature coronary artery disease

- **Treatment**
  - Surgical removal of the pituitary tumor
  - Pharmacologic therapy with somatostatin analogs or dopamine agonists

- **Pearl**

Carney syndrome is a rare disorder involving any 3 of the following: growth hormone–secreting pituitary tumor, cardiac or cutaneous myxoma, Sertoli cell tumors, cutaneous hyperpigmentation, or pigmented nodular adrenocortical disease.

Reference

Colao A et al: Growth hormone and the heart. Clin Endocrinol (Oxf) 2001;54:137.

Adrenal Insufficiency & the Heart

- **Essentials of Diagnosis**
  - Inability to increase cortisol to more than 20 mg/dL in response to synthetic adrenocorticotropic hormone (ACTH) during rapid ACTH stimulation testing
  - Orthostatic hypotension, salt wasting, and hyperkalemia in primary adrenal insufficiency (Addison disease)
  - Hyponatremia in both primary and secondary (pituitary) adrenal insufficiency
  - Elevated ACTH in Addison disease

- **Differential Diagnosis**
  - Other causes of orthostatic hypotension
  - Other causes of hypovolemic shock
  - Other causes of hyperkalemia, hyponatremia, hypercalcemia, hypoglycemia, and acidosis

- **Treatment**
  - Hydrocortisone 100 mg intravenously (IV) every 6–8 hours acutely
  - Saline and glucose IV
  - Treatment of precipitating infection
  - Long-term adrenal hormone replacement

- **Pearl**

Secondary adrenal insufficiency occurs in about one third of critically ill patients.

Reference

Zolga GP, Marik P: Endocrine and metabolic dysfunction syndromes in the critically ill. Crit Care Clin 2001;17:25.

Cushing Syndrome

- **Essentials of Diagnosis**
    - Excess cortisol in the circulation
    - Central obesity
    - Hypertension
    - Hyperlipidemia
    - Hyperglycemia

- **Differential Diagnosis**
    - Pseudo-Cushing syndrome: patients appear cushingoid but have normal screening laboratory tests
    - Other causes of obesity, hypertension, hyperlipidemia, and hyperglycemia

- **Treatment**
    - Surgical removal of the pituitary, adrenal, or ectopic tumor
    - If surgery is not feasible, adrenolytic pharmacologic agents can be used

- **Pearl**

Remember that exogenous steroid use can cause Cushing syndrome.

Reference

Boscaro M et al: The diagnosis of Cushing's syndrome: Atypical presentations and laboratory shortcomings. Arch Intern Med 2000;160:3045.

Diabetic Cardiomyopathy

■ Essentials of Diagnosis
- Diabetes mellitus type 2, especially in women
- Unexplained heart failure without hypertension or large epicardial coronary artery disease
- Left ventricular hypertrophy with systolic and diastolic dysfunction by echocardiography

■ Differential Diagnosis
- Atherosclerotic cardiovascular disease with silent infarction
- Hypertensive heart disease
- Other causes of heart failure

■ Treatment
- Tight control of blood glucose (hemoglobin A1c <7.0%)
- Angiotensin-converting enzyme inhibitors titrated to achieve blood pressure less than 130/85 mm Hg
- Correction of dyslipidemia
- Other treatment for heart failure as needed

■ Pearl

Beta-blockers are often underutilized in diabetes because of the fear that glycemic control will be difficult and they will mask symptoms of hypoglycemia. However, beta-blockers are usually more effective in diabetic patients than in nondiabetic patients, and cardioselective agents do not upset glycemic control or hypoglycemia perception appreciably.

Reference

Sakamoto K et al: Mechanism of impaired left ventricular wall motion in the diabetic heart without coronary artery disease. Diabetes Care 1998;21:2123.

Hyperaldosteronism, Primary

- ■ Essentials of Diagnosis
  - • Hypertension due to sodium and water retention
  - • Hypokalemia and alkalosis
  - • Suppressed plasma renin and elevated aldosterone
  - • Imaging results showing adrenal adenoma or hyperplasia

- ■ Differential Diagnosis
  - • Other causes of hypertension (primary aldosteronism accounts for 10–20% of hypertensive patients referred to hypertension clinics)
  - • Other causes of hypokalemia

- ■ Treatment
  - • Surgical resection of adenoma
  - • Aldosterone antagonists for hyperplasia—spironolactone, amiloride, and calcium channel blockers

- ■ Pearl

Although the most common cause of hypokalemia in hypertensive patients is potassium-wasting diuretic use, a serum potassium level less than 3.0 mmol/L in a patient taking diuretics should arouse suspicion of primary hyperaldosteronism.

Reference

Young WF Jr: Primary aldosteronism: A common and curable form of hypertension. Cardiol Rev 1999;7:2107.

Hyperlipidemia (Lipid Disorders)

■ **Essentials of Diagnosis**
- Total serum cholesterol greater than 200 mg/dL in 2 samples at least 2 weeks apart
- Low-density lipoprotein (LDL) cholesterol greater than 100 mg/dL
- High-density lipoprotein (HDL) cholesterol less than 40 mg/dL
- Triglycerides greater than 200 mg/dL

■ **Differential Diagnosis**
- Hypothyroidism increases LDL cholesterol
- Nonfasting state increases triglycerides
- Diabetes increases triglycerides, reduces HDL cholesterol
- Alcohol increases triglycerides
- Oral contraceptives increase triglycerides
- Nephrotic syndrome increases LDL cholesterol and triglycerides
- Renal failure increases LDL cholesterol and triglycerides
- Primary biliary cirrhosis increases LDL cholesterol
- Acute hepatitis increases triglycerides
- Obesity increases triglycerides

■ **Treatment**

Nonpharmacologic
- Exercise, weight loss, low-fat diet (cholesterol <200 mg/d, fat <30% of total calories, saturated fat <7% of total calories), and high-fiber diet

Pharmacologic
- Bile acid sequestrants: cholestyramine, colestipol, colesevelam
- Intestinal endothelium blockers: ezetimibe
- Fibric acid derivatives: gemfibrozil, clofibrate, fenofibrate
- Nicotinic acid
- Hepatic 3-methylglutaryl coenzyme A reductase inhibitors: atorvastatin, pravastatin, simvastatin

■ **Pearl**

Eruptive xanthomas are characteristic of high triglyceride levels, whereas tendon xanthomas (ie, Achilles) are characteristic of high LDL cholesterol levels. Xanthelasma are nonspecific and can be found in individuals without lipid disorders.

Reference

Expert Panel on Detection, Evaluation, and Treatment of High Blood Cholesterol in Adults: Executive summary of the third report of the National Cholesterol Education Program (NCEP) Expert Panel on Detection, Evaluation, and Treatment of High Blood Cholesterol in Adults (Adult Treatment Panel III). JAMA 2001;285:2486.

Hyperparathyroidism & the Heart

- ■ Essentials of Diagnosis
  - Elevated serum calcium due to parathyroid hormone excess
  - Valvular sclerosis and left ventricular hypertrophy
  - Electrocardiogram (ECG) exhibits shortened ST segment and reduced QT interval
  - Acute hypercalcemia can cause hypertension, bradycardia, and heart block

- ■ Differential Diagnosis
  - Other causes of hypercalcemia without parathyroid hormone excess
  - Valvular sclerosis from atherosclerosis or rheumatic disease
  - Other causes of hypertension and left ventricular hypertrophy

- ■ Treatment
  - Parathyroidectomy is the definitive treatment
  - Pharmacologic treatment with biphosphates, pamidronate, risedronate, and estrogen in postmenopausal women is less effective
  - Acute hypercalcemia is treated with saline infusion plus furosemide. Thiazide diuretics are contraindicated.

- ■ Pearl

A shortened QT interval corrected for heart rate (QTc) is the most reliable ECG index of hypercalcemia (<0.39 in men, <0.41 in women). The QTc interval is inversely proportional to the serum calcium up to serum calcium levels of 16 mg/dL. At greater calcium levels, the T wave widens, increasing the QTc.

Reference

Piovesan A et al: Left ventricular hypertrophy in primary hyperparathyroidism. Effects of successful parathyroidectomy. Clin Endocrinol (Oxf) 1999;50:321.

Hyperthyroid Heart Disease

- ■ Essentials of Diagnosis
  - Palpitations, dyspnea, chest pain
  - Atrial fibrillation, tachycardia
  - Hyperreflexia, tremor
  - Stare, lid lag, and lid retraction due to high catecholamines
  - Depressed thyroid-stimulating hormone and high thyroxine levels
  - Goiter and exophthalmos in Graves disease

- ■ Differential Diagnosis
  - Anxiety disorder
  - Factitious or iatrogenic thyrotoxicosis
  - Angina, atrial fibrillation, and other signs without thyrotoxicosis

- ■ Treatment
  - Beta-blockers to reduce heart rate and improve symptoms; propranolol is preferred because it blocks peripheral conversion of T4 to T3
  - Thionamides to block thyroid hormone release and prevent synthesis
  - Radioactive iodine ablation
  - Subtotal thyroidectomy in selected cases

- ■ Pearl

Most patients with congestive heart failure in association with thyrotoxicosis have underlying cardiac disease. Pure high-output heart failure is rare.

Reference

Klein I, Ojamaa K: Thyroid hormone and the cardiovascular system. N Engl J Med 2001;344:501.

Hypothyroid Heart Disease

- **Essentials of Diagnosis**
  - Weakness, weight gain, cold intolerance
  - Reduced exercise tolerance, dyspnea on exertion
  - Pleural and pericardial effusions, edema, anasarca
  - Bradycardia, hypothermia, mild hypertension
  - Goiter, delayed reflexes, myxedema coma
  - Elevated thyroid-stimulating hormone and reduced thyroxine levels
  - Hyperlipidemia and premature atherosclerosis

- **Differential Diagnosis**
  - Congestive heart failure due to other causes
  - Other causes of effusions and edema
  - Hyperlipidemia and atherosclerosis without hypothyroidism

- **Treatment**
  - Thyroid hormone replacement, which must be given slowly to older patients or those suspected of having coronary artery disease, to prevent exacerbation of angina and precipitation of myocardial infarction
  - Coronary revascularization should be considered before thyroid replacement therapy in high-risk patients

- **Pearl**

True congestive heart failure rarely occurs in hypothyroidism because the decrease in cardiac output is proportional to the decrease in metabolic demand.

Reference

Tielens ET et al: Changes in cardiac function at rest before and after treatment in primary hypothyroidism. Am J Cardiol 2000;85:376.

Metabolic Syndrome & the Heart

- **Essentials of Diagnosis**
  - Truncal obesity
  - Insulin resistance with fasting hyperglycemia
  - Elevated triglycerides and LDL cholesterol
  - Hypertension
  - Hyperuricemia
  - Premature coronary artery disease

- **Differential Diagnosis**
  - Other causes of premature coronary artery disease
  - Other causes of hypertension
  - Other causes of obesity

- **Treatment**
  - Dietary modification, weight loss
  - Oral hypoglycemic agents, insulin sensitizers, and insulin
  - Pharmacologic treatment of hypertension with angiotensin-converting enzyme inhibitors or angiotensin-receptor blockers to less than 130/80 mm Hg
  - Pharmacologic lipid-lowering therapy to LDL cholesterol less than 100 mg/dL

- **Pearl**

Although these patients may not meet criteria for frank diabetes, they are at high risk for developing premature cardiovascular disease.

Reference

Vega GL: Obesity, the metabolic syndrome, and cardiovascular disease. Am Heart J 2001;142:1108.

10

General Cardiology

Ankylosing Spondylitis & the Heart

- ■ Essentials of Diagnosis
  - Characteristic lumbar spine and sacroiliac arthritis; positive HLA-B27 assay
  - Aortic root sclerosis and dilation, leaflet thickening, and subaortic bump on echocardiography
  - Aortic regurgitation

- ■ Differential Diagnosis
  - Other causes of aortic valve disease
  - Other connective tissue diseases

- ■ Treatment
  - Specific anti-inflammatory pharmacotherapy
  - Antibiotic prophylaxis
  - Vasodilators or surgery for more severe aortic regurgitation

- ■ Pearl

In young men (age <40 years) with significant aortic regurgitation, ankylosing spondylitis should be considered, especially if they have any back complaints or signs.

Reference

Roldan CA et al: Aortic root disease and valve disease associated with ankylosing spondylitis. J Am Coll Cardiol 1998;32:1397.

Athlete's Heart

- **Essentials of Diagnosis**
  - History of athletic training and performance
  - Enhanced exercise ability (maximum O_2 uptake >40 mL/kg/min)
  - Resting bradycardia
  - Increased left ventricular mass by echocardiography

- **Differential Diagnosis**
  - Pathologic left ventricular volume increase (ie, dilated cardiomyopathy)
  - Pathologic left ventricular hypertrophy, especially hypertrophic cardiomyopathy
  - Pathologic bradycardia
  - Coronary artery disease

- **Treatment**
  - For symptomatic bradycardias with orthostatic intolerance, reduce or stop isotonic training
  - Cessation of training during viral illnesses reduces the incidence of myocarditis

- **Pearl**

Right and left ventricular enlargement in trained athletes can lead to pseudomyocardial infarct patterns on the electrocardiogram (ECG).

Reference

Pellicia A et al: The upper limit of physiologic cardiac hypertrophy in highly trained elite athletes. N Engl J Med 1991;324:295.

Carcinoid & the Heart

- ■ Essentials of Diagnosis
  - Computed tomography (CT) or other imaging of neuroendocrine tumor(s) in the gut, with possible liver or pulmonary metastases
  - Elevated 5-hydroxyindoleacetic acid in the urine
  - Cardiac auscultatory evidence of tricuspid regurgitation or pulmonic stenosis
  - Echocardiographic evidence of thickened tricuspid or pulmonary valves

- ■ Differential Diagnosis
  - Other causes of pulmonic stenosis, tricuspid regurgitation, and right-heart failure
  - Consumption of serotonin-rich foods can give false-positive urine screening tests

- ■ Treatment
  - Surgical removal of the tumor if it has not metastasized
  - Somatostatin therapy to shrink metastases
  - Valve replacement in selected patients with slowly progressive disease

- ■ Pearl

Carcinoid syndrome is the only condition that causes thickening and dysfunction of both right-heart valves.

Reference

Ganim RB, Norton JA: Recent advances in carcinoid pathogenesis, diagnosis and management. Surg Oncol 2000;9:173.

Cardiac Contusion/Blunt Trauma

- **Essentials of Diagnosis**
  - May range from minor myocardial bruise to cardiac rupture
  - Chest pain not responding to nitrates may suggest contusion
  - Evidence of other injuries, such as rib fracture or impression of the steering wheel on the anterior chest wall
  - Inadequate hemodynamic response to appropriate resuscitative measures
  - Clinically significant myocardial injury with intact pericardium presents as cardiac tamponade
  - When the pericardium is not intact, extrapericardial bleeding causes hypovolemic shock
  - Valvular dysfunction secondary to tear or rupture may not cause acute symptoms, but later may present as heart failure
  - Hemodynamically stable patients with normal ECG require no additional testing
  - ECG abnormalities, most commonly nonspecific repolarization changes, consistently accompany contusion
  - Cardiac enzymes may be elevated but do not have prognostic value; abnormal ECG is the best predictor of complications

- **Differential Diagnosis**
  - ECG changes secondary to coronary artery disease
  - Noncardiac intrathoracic trauma
  - Cardiac enzyme elevation secondary to noncardiac trauma

- **Treatment**
  - Pharmacologic agents for ventricular arrhythmia
  - Invasive hemodynamic monitoring in hemodynamically unstable patients
  - Monitoring for patients with minor trauma but abnormal ECG
  - Pericardiocentesis for patients with cardiac tamponade
  - Definitive treatment in critical patients: thoracotomy (or sternotomy) and appropriate surgical repair

- **Pearl**

Patients with suspected chest trauma and abnormal ECG must be monitored in the hospital for arrhythmia.

Reference

Sybrandy KC et al: Diagnosing cardiac contusion: Old wisdom and new insights. Heart 2003;89:485.

Cocaine-Induced Cardiovascular Disease

- **Essentials of Diagnosis**
  - Chest pain and myocardial infarction
  - Features of congestive heart failure secondary to cocaine cardiomyopathy
  - Hypertension
  - Positive history or urine drug screen for cocaine (history of cocaine use may be denied and urine drug screen may be negative)
  - ECG is often nonspecific (non–Q-wave infarction is more common than Q-wave infarction in cocaine users)

- **Differential Diagnosis**
  - Atherosclerotic coronary artery disease
  - Spontaneous coronary artery spasm

- **Treatment**
  - Nitrates, alpha-adrenoreceptor blockers, and verapamil for acute ischemia
  - Aspirin
  - Thrombolytic therapy in acute ST-elevation myocardial infarction
  - Beta-blockers should be avoided
  - Emergent coronary angiography and primary angioplasty may be used as alternative means of establishing perfusion, particularly if diagnosis is uncertain because of early repolarization
  - Lidocaine should be used cautiously because it lowers the seizure threshold

- **Pearl**

The differential diagnosis of young patients with the presentation of acute coronary syndrome should include cocaine-induced myocardial infarction. Avoid beta-blockers in this group unless the tachycardia cannot be controlled by alternative means.

Reference

Kloner RA, Rezkalla SH: Cocaine and the heart. N Engl J Med 2003;348:487.

Contrast Nephropathy

- **Essentials of Diagnosis**
  - Hypoxic tubular injury due to vasoconstriction with release of free oxygen radicals is the likely mechanism
  - Increase in serum creatinine of greater than 50% represents clinically important acute renal failure
  - Major risk factors are prior renal insufficiency and diabetes mellitus
  - Minor risk factors are congestive heart failure, dehydration, hypotension, hypoxia, large amount of contrast, ionic and high osmolar contrast, repeated examinations at short intervals, and abdominal examination; other risk factors may include age, smoking, hypercholesterolemia, and use of non-steroidal anti-inflammatory drugs
  - The peak in serum creatinine occurs within 2–5 days after exposure and returns to baseline in most cases

- **Differential Diagnosis**
  - Atheroembolic renal failure
  - Pre-renal azotemia secondary to low cardiac output

- **Prevention & Treatment**
  - Adequate hydration (0.45% normal saline at 1 mL/kg/h for 12 hours before and 12 hours after the procedure) is the most important therapy for preventing contrast nephropathy in high-risk patients
  - N-acetylcysteine 600 mg orally twice daily before and after administration of the contrast agent is a useful adjunct for prevention in high-risk patients
  - Fenoldopam (0.1 µg/kg/min), the dopamine-1 receptor agonist, is a useful adjunct in high-risk patients
  - Iodixanol, an iso-osmolar contrast agent, is useful for prevention in high-risk patients
  - Once contrast nephropathy occurs, treatment is similar to that for any other cause of acute renal insufficiency; most patients improve spontaneously with conservative management, but a few may require temporary dialysis. Need for long-term dialysis purely for contrast nephropathy is rare.

- **Pearl**

Prevention is better than cure. Identify high-risk patients and use the outlined strategies to prevent contrast nephropathy.

Reference

Lindholt JS: Radiocontrast induced nephropathy. Eur J Vasc Endovasc Surg 2003;25:296.

Digitalis Toxicity

■ Essentials of Diagnosis

- May occur in 30% of patients hospitalized for heart failure
- Common clinical features include nausea, vomiting, anorexia, malaise, drowsiness, headache, insomnia, altered color vision, or arrhythmia
- Almost all known cardiac arrhythmias may be caused by digitalis toxicity
- Common arrhythmias due to digitalis toxicity include premature ventricular beats, junctional tachycardia, second- or third-degree heart block, and paroxysmal atrial tachycardia with block
- Toxicity is facilitated by hypokalemia; severe digoxin toxicity causes hyperkalemia secondary to paralysis of Na^+/K^+ exchange pump
- Diuretics cause hypokalemia and thus facilitate digitalis toxicity

■ Differential Diagnosis

- Arrhythmias secondary to underlying heart disease
- Gastrointestinal disorders

■ Treatment

- Reversal of symptoms or cessation of arrhythmia occurs after withdrawal of digoxin for 48 hours
- Ventricular arrhythmia may require phenytoin or lidocaine
- Antidigoxin immunotherapy may be used, particularly if hyperkalemia is present

■ Pearl

Serum levels of digoxin do not correlate well with signs and symptoms of digitalis toxicity. Digitalis toxicity is largely a clinical diagnosis.

Reference

Rathore SS et al: Association of serum digoxin concentration and outcomes in patients with heart failure. JAMA 2003;289:871.

Friedreich Ataxia, Cardiac Manifestations

- ■ Essentials of Diagnosis
  - • Neurologic symptoms usually precede cardiac symptoms
  - • Frequently associated with concentric hypertrophic cardiomyopathy (abnormalities of the gene that encodes fataxin, a protein expressed in the normal heart that may play a role in causing hypertrophy)
  - • Dilated cardiomyopathy occurs rarely
  - • Echocardiography shows left ventricular hypertrophy; ECG may not show changes of hypertrophy despite the echocardiographic evidence
  - • Widespread T-wave inversion is detected on the ECG
  - • Atrial fibrillation, atrial flutter, and ventricular tachycardia may occur in the presence of dilated cardiomyopathy; ventricular tachyarrhythmias are not associated with hypertrophic cardiomyopathy

- ■ Differential Diagnosis
  - • Hypertrophic cardiomyopathy (asymmetric septal hypertrophy may occur, but myocardial fiber disarray as described in genetic hypertrophic cardiomyopathy is rare)

- ■ Treatment
  - • Symptomatic management of arrhythmias
  - • Pharmacologic management of heart failure

- ■ Pearl

Hypertrophic cardiomyopathy is common in Friedreich ataxia. This cardiomyopathy is different from genetic hypertrophic cardiomyopathy even if there is a left ventricular outflow tract gradient. Dilated cardiomyopathy carries a very poor prognosis.

Reference

Weidemann F et al: Quantification of regional right and left ventricular function by ultrasonic strain rate and strain indexes in Friedreich's ataxia. Am J Cardiol 2003;91:622.

Heart Disease in Pregnancy

- **Essentials of Diagnosis**
  - Pregnancy
  - History of heart disease
  - Symptoms, signs, and echocardiographic evidence of heart disease

- **Differential Diagnosis**
  - Symptoms from increased cardiac output in normal pregnancy (eg, fatigue, dyspnea on exertion, reduced exercise tolerance)
  - Symptoms from reduced peripheral resistance in normal pregnancy (eg, dizziness, presyncope, orthostatic intolerance)
  - Symptoms from compression of the inferior vena cava by the gravid uterus (eg, orthopnea, chest pressure)
  - Signs of increased blood volume in normal pregnancy (eg, jugular venous distention, enlarged left ventricular impulse, right ventricular lift, palpable pulmonary artery impulse, increased intensity of the first heart sound, systolic ejection murmur at the left sternal border, cervical venous hum)

- **Treatment**
  - Avoid unnecessary drug treatment of cardiac conditions, especially in the first trimester. Unsafe drugs include angiotensin-converting enzyme inhibitors, angiotensin-receptor blockers, amiodarone, calcium channel blockers, and warfarin.
  - Heart failure can be treated with digoxin, hydralazine, diuretics, and nitrates
  - Arrhythmias can be treated with digoxin, adenosine, quinidine, procainamide, lidocaine, and beta-blockers
  - Necessary anticoagulation for patients with prosthetic valves: heparin for the first trimester, then warfarin until 36–38 weeks, then heparin again until 4–6 hours after delivery
  - Percutaneous valvuloplasty (mitral or pulmonic) is feasible during pregnancy, as is cardiac surgery not involving heart-lung bypass, which often causes fetal wastage
  - The preferred method of delivery is vaginal with regional anesthesia; antibiotic prophylaxis should be given when indicated

- **Pearl**

The normal physiologic changes of pregnancy reduce the intensity of the murmurs associated with aortic and mitral regurgitation and hypertrophic cardiomyopathy.

Reference

Gibson GJ et al: Changes in hemodynamics, ventricular remodeling, and ventricular contractility during normal pregnancy: A longitudinal study. Obstet Gynecol 1997;89:957.

Hypotension Complicating Hemodialysis

- **Essentials of Diagnosis**
  - Marked decrease (>30 mm Hg systolic) in blood pressure during dialysis
  - Symptoms of decreased cerebral perfusion

- **Differential Diagnosis**
  - Pericardial effusion due to uremia or other causes
  - Left ventricular diastolic dysfunction due to hypertrophy
  - Autonomic dysfunction, often due to diabetes
  - Myocardial ischemia (may be produced by hypotension also)
  - Overzealous use of antihypertensive agents
  - Cardiac arrhythmias
  - Severe left ventricular systolic dysfunction
  - Low dry weight of patient
  - Decreased plasma osmolarity
  - Splanchnic vasodilation due to a large meal
  - Characteristics of the dialysate (eg, acetate)

- **Treatment**
  - Identify and remove pericardial fluid
  - Identify and treat myocardial ischemia
  - Carefully adjust antihypertensive medications
  - Prevent cardiac arrhythmias
  - Treat heart failure
  - Decrease fluid removal in patients with low dry weight
  - Adjust sodium in dialysate to greater than 135 mmol/L to prevent hypo-osmolarity
  - Use cooled bicarbonate dialysate
  - Administer vasoconstrictors in refractory cases

- **Pearl**

ECG monitoring during dialysis may reveal myocardial ischemia, arrhythmias, or inappropriate bradycardia.

Reference

Schreiber MJ Jr: Clinical case-based approach to understanding intradialytic hypotension. Am J Kidney Dis 2001;38:S37.

Inherited Neuromuscular Disease & the Heart

- ■ Essentials of Diagnosis
    - Evidence of progressive muscle wasting and weakness
    - Dilated cardiomyopathy
    - Conduction abnormalities
    - Arrhythmias
    - Nonspecific ECG abnormalities
    - Specific genetic diagnosis of a muscular dystrophy

- ■ Differential Diagnosis
    - Cardiomyopathy from other causes with muscle atrophy and weakness from inactivity (cardiac cachexia)
    - Conduction, rhythm, and ECG abnormalities from other causes

- ■ Treatment
    - Therapy as indicated for heart failure
    - Pacemaker or implantable cardioverter-defibrillator as indicated
    - Antiarrhythmic drug therapy as appropriate

- ■ Pearl

Cardiac transplantation is usually not an option in these muscular dystrophies, such as Duchenne, because the progressive and profound muscular deterioration leads to respiratory failure and death. However, in milder forms such as Becker muscular dystrophy, cardiac transplantation is feasible.

Reference

Politano L et al: Development of cardiomyopathy in female carriers of Duchenne and Becker muscular dystrophies. JAMA 1996;275:1335.

Left Atrial Myxoma

- **Essentials of Diagnosis**
  - Symptoms of valvular dysfunction such as dyspnea
  - Thromboemboli
  - Constitutional symptoms (eg, fever, arthralgias, weight loss)
  - Tumor plop sound in early diastole; mitral systolic or diastolic murmurs
  - Echocardiographic evidence of characteristic cardiac mass

- **Differential Diagnosis**
  - Cardiac thrombus
  - Vegetations
  - Flail or prolapsing leaflets
  - Mitral valve disease

- **Treatment**
  - Expeditious surgical removal
  - Cardiac transplantation

- **Pearl**

The cardiac physical findings of left atrial myxoma can resemble rheumatic mitral stenosis.

Reference

Schaff HV, Mullany CJ: Surgery for cardiac myxomas. Semin Thorac Cardiovasc Surg 2000;12:77.

Marfan Syndrome

- **Essentials of Diagnosis**
  - Autosomal dominant disorder (frequency of 1 per 10,000) with multisystem involvement
  - Affects the skeleton (long thin extremities), eye (ectopia lentis), and the cardiovascular system (aortic aneurysms) from mutation in a gene on chromosome 15 that encodes fibrillin
  - Mitral valve prolapse secondary to redundancy of the leaflets and the chordae occurs in 60–80%
  - Mitral regurgitation becomes severe in 25% of patients
  - Aortic root dilatation and aortic regurgitation occur
  - Dissection of the aorta occurs with increasing frequency at a diameter of 55 mm (family history of dissection increases the risk at 50 mm)
  - Pregnancy increases the risk of dissection, particularly in the third trimester; risk is low if the root diameter is less than 40 mm

- **Differential Diagnosis**
  - Homocystinuria
  - Ehlers-Danlos syndrome
  - Familial aortic aneurysm

- **Treatment**
  - Endocarditis prophylaxis
  - Restriction from heavy weight lifting and contact sports
  - Beta-blockers to prevent or delay aortic root dilatation (recommended, but efficacy is not established)
  - Surgical replacement of aorta with preservation of native aortic valve (either prophylactic at aortic root diameter of >50 mm, or treatment for dissection)
  - In pregnancy, consider surgery at 40–50 mm aortic root diameter
  - Mitral valve surgery if mitral regurgitation is severe and patient is symptomatic

- **Pearl**

Not all patients with dissection of the aorta associated with Marfan syndrome complain of severe chest pain; take vague complaints seriously and investigate.

Reference

Dean JC: Management of Marfan syndrome. Heart 2002;88:97.

Metabolic Abnormalities & Cardiovascular Disease

- ■ Essentials of Diagnosis
  - • Hyponatremia is common in advanced heart failure; diuretics may also play a role
  - • Hypokalemia is also common with use of diuretics; hypokalemia increases the risk of ventricular arrhythmia particularly with digitalis toxicity; ECG may have prominent U waves; extreme hypokalemia may lead to cardiac arrest
  - • Hyperkalemia causes peaked T waves, absent P waves, and QRS prolongation; more severe degree leads to sine-wave pattern or asystole
  - • Hypocalcemia prolongs QT interval; hypercalcemia shortens QT interval
  - • Hypocalcemia and hypophosphatemia, when prolonged, may cause cardiomyopathy
  - • Hypomagnesemia may cause refractory hypokalemia and hypocalcemia; it also may cause ventricular arrhythmias

- ■ Differential Diagnosis
  - • Hypokalemia and hypomagnesemia may be caused by diuretics or gastrointestinal losses
  - • Angiotensin-converting enzyme inhibitors and spironolactone may cause hyperkalemia

- ■ Treatment
  - • Identify and treat the underlying cause
  - • For hypokalemia and hypomagnesemia, provide intravenous (IV) or oral replacement
  - • Severe hyperkalemia is a cardiac emergency; use IV calcium chloride or gluconate for cardioprotection, IV insulin/glucose and/or bicarbonate to shift the potassium into the cell, sodium polystyrene sulfonate or diuretic to lower body potassium subacutely, and dialysis if necessary

- ■ Pearl

Unexplained orthostatic hypotension may be caused by hypokalemia.

Reference

Cohn JN et al: New guidelines for potassium replacement in clinical practice: A contemporary review by the National Council on Potassium in Clinical Practice. Arch Intern Med 2000;160:2429.

Metastatic Tumors to the Heart

- ■ Essentials of Diagnosis
  - Evidence of tumors elsewhere in the body, especially bronchogenic carcinoma, breast cancer, lymphoma, and leukemia
  - Positive imaging study for characteristic cardiac masses
  - Positive biopsy of cardiac masses

- ■ Differential Diagnosis
  - Primary cardiac tumors: metastatic tumors are 50 times more common
  - Melanoma has a high predilection for cardiac metastases (half of cases)
  - Thrombus: renal cell carcinoma may grow up the inferior vena cava and mimic thrombus in the right atrium
  - Vegetations; flail or prolapsing cardiac valves
  - Pericardial cysts
  - Giant aneurysm of the coronary artery
  - Diaphragmatic hernia can mimic left atrial mass on transthoracic echocardiography
  - Lipomatous infiltration
  - Normal anatomic variants: Chiari network, eustachian valve, septum spurium, thebesian valve, left superior pulmonary vein, atrial septal aneurysm

- ■ Treatment
  - Pharmacologic therapy is usually disappointing
  - Radiation therapy can prolong life
  - Surgery is definitive therapy, but is rarely considered unless cure of the primary tumor is highly likely
  - Pericardiocentesis, percutaneous pericardiostomy, and partial pericardiectomy may be required because of pericardial tamponade. If surgery is not feasible, sclerosing agents such as doxycycline can be instilled to prevent recurrences of cardiac tamponade

- ■ Pearl

On echocardiography or other cardiac imaging, masses that cross anatomic planes (ie, from myocardium to pericardium or to endocardium) are likely to be tumors.

Reference

Keefe DL: Cardiovascular emergencies in the cancer patient. Semin Oncol 2000;27:244.

Mixed Connective Tissue Disease & the Heart

- **Essentials of Diagnosis**
  - Raynaud phenomenon, sclerodactyly
  - Myopathy with high titers of ribonucleoprotein antibodies
  - Pericarditis, pulmonary hypertension

- **Differential Diagnosis**
  - Other connective tissue diseases
  - Other causes of cardiac disease

- **Treatment**
  - Specific anti-inflammatory pharmacotherapy
  - Calcium channel blockers for pulmonary hypertension

- **Pearl**

Up to one third of patients with mixed connective tissue disease have mitral valve prolapse.

Reference

Rebollar-Gonzalez V et al: Cardiac conduction disturbances in mixed connective tissue disease. Rev Invest Clin 2001;53:330.

Obesity & Heart Disease

■ Essentials of Diagnosis

- Body mass index greater than 30 kg/m^2
- Increased left ventricular mass by imaging in the absence of hypertension or diabetes
- Heart failure and cardiac arrhythmias are common

■ Differential Diagnosis

- Coronary artery disease
- Dilated cardiomyopathy
- Hypertrophic cardiomyopathy
- Diabetic cardiomyopathy

■ Treatment

- Weight loss via diet, exercise, approved drugs, or surgery
- Assessment and treatment of comorbid conditions such as hyperlipidemia
- Indicated treatment for heart failure or arrhythmias

■ Pearl

The risk of cardiovascular disease associated with obesity is strongest in those of European descent. In many other ethnic groups, this risk association is much less apparent. One possible explanation is that physical fitness despite obesity (eg, sumo wrestlers) reduces cardiovascular disease morbidity and mortality.

Reference

Stevens J et al: The effect of age on the association between body mass index and mortality. N Engl J Med 1998;338:1.

Polymyositis/Dermatomyositis & the Heart

- **Essentials of Diagnosis**
  - Muscle weakness, characteristic skin lesions
  - Arrhythmias or conduction disturbances and myocarditis
  - Pericarditis, coronary arteritis, valve disease

- **Differential Diagnosis**
  - Other connective tissue diseases
  - Other causes of cardiac disease

- **Treatment**
  - Specific anti-inflammatory pharmacotherapy
  - Specific cardiac therapy as indicated

- **Pearl**

Active myositis often parallels myocarditis, so when a patient presents with both, think of polymyositis/dermatomyositis.

Reference

Spiera R, Kagen L: Extramuscular manifestations in idiopathic inflammatory myopathies. Curr Opin Rheumatol 1998;10:556.

Primary Tumors of the Heart (Excluding Myxoma)

- Essentials of Diagnosis
  - Positive imaging study for characteristic cardiac masses
  - Positive biopsy of cardiac masses

- Differential Diagnosis
  - Metastatic tumors
  - Thrombus
  - Nonbacterial thrombolic endocarditis
  - Vegetations from infective endocarditis
  - Flail or prolapsing valve leaflets
  - Giant aneurysm of the coronary artery
  - Pericardial cyst
  - Diaphragmatic hernia
  - Lipomatous cardiac infiltration
  - Normal anatomic variants: Chiari network, eustachian valve, septum spurium, thebesian valve, left superior pulmonary vein, atrial septal aneurysm

- Treatment
  - Pharmacologic therapy is adjunctive for specific tumors
  - Radiation therapy is adjunctive for specific situations
  - Surgery can be curative or used to reduce symptoms
  - Cardiac transplantation is an alternative for unresectable tumors

- Pearl

Most primary cardiac tumors (75–80%) are benign and therefore potentially curable.

Reference

Vaughan CJ et al: Tumors and the heart: Molecular genetic advances. Curr Opin Cardiol 2001;16:195.

Pulmonary Embolism

- ■ Essentials of Diagnosis
  - Seen in immobilized patients (eg, after surgery) and in patients with congestive heart failure, malignancies, pelvic trauma, and deep venous thrombosis
  - Otherwise unexplained dyspnea, tachypnea, or chest pain
  - Clinical, ECG, or echocardiographic evidence of acute cor pulmonale
  - Elevated plasma D-dimer enzyme-linked immunosorbent assay
  - Positive spiral chest CT scan with contrast
  - High-probability ventilation-perfusion lung scan or high-probability perfusion lung scan with a normal chest radiograph
  - Positive venous ultrasound for thrombus in the legs, with a convincing clinical history and a suggestive lung scan
  - Diagnostic pulmonary angiogram

- ■ Differential Diagnosis
  - Pneumonia
  - Myocardial infarction
  - Pulmonary disorder with pleurisy
  - Respiratory distress secondary to pulmonary edema, asthma, or pleural effusion
  - Early sepsis
  - Psychogenic hyperventilation

- ■ Treatment
  - Acute anticoagulation with heparin for several days, with warfarin instituted concurrently and continuing for 6 months
  - Thrombolytic therapy in patients with hemodynamic compromise (no proven effect on mortality)
  - Intravenous filter placement in the inferior vena cava for patients who are not candidates for anticoagulation (because of bleeding) or are unresponsive to anticoagulation

- ■ Pearl

Ten percent of pulmonary emboli originate from upper-extremity veins.

Reference

Dalen JE: Pulmonary embolism: What have we learned since Virchow? Natural history, pathophysiology, and diagnosis. Chest 2002;122:1440.

Radiation Heart Disease

- **Essentials of Diagnosis**
    - History of mediastinal radiation therapy, usually for Hodgkin disease
    - Pericarditis early or within 1 year or more
    - Cardiomyopathy, especially if treated with anthracyclines also
    - Coronary artery disease after a 3- to 20-year latency period
    - Valvular regurgitation; occasionally stenosis
    - Heart block; occasionally tachyarrhythmias

- **Differential Diagnosis**
    - Pericarditis from other causes, especially hypothyroidism (thyroid in field)
    - Cardiomyopathy from other causes, especially anthracyclines
    - Coronary artery disease from other causes
    - Valvular heart disease from other causes
    - Cardiac arrhythmias from other causes

- **Prevention & Treatment**

    Prevention
    - Modern radiation therapy reduces the risk; steroids can prevent fibrosis

    Treatment
    - Pericarditis: treat in the usual fashion, but pericardiectomy is more frequently required
    - Coronary artery disease: angioplasty is less successful than bypass surgery, but the risk of bypass surgery is increased by lung or right ventricular damage, and sometimes the internal thoracic arteries have been damaged and other conduits are necessary
    - Valvular disease: surgery is often complicated by pericardial and coronary artery disease
    - Heart block: A-V sequential pacing is recommended because the ventricles are often stiff

- **Pearl**

    Radiation therapy should be considered a cardiac disease risk factor; it is imperative to reduce other risk factors as much as possible.

Reference

Glauzmann C et al: Cardiac risk after mediastinal irradiation for Hodgkin's disease. Radiother Oncol 1998;46:51.

Renal Dysfunction in Heart Failure

■ **Essentials of Diagnosis**

- Congestive heart failure with elevated serum creatinine and blood urea nitrogen

■ **Differential Diagnosis**

- Primary renal disease such as renovascular disease, obstructive uropathy, or urinary tract infection
- Drug-induced renal dysfunction: non-steroidal anti-inflammatory drugs, allopurinol, angiotensin-converting enzyme inhibitors
- Volume depletion from aggressive use of diuretics

■ **Treatment**

- Stop unnecessary drugs
- Carefully adjust dosage of angiotensin-converting enzyme inhibitors
- Carefully adjust diuretic dosage
- Maximize beta-blocker therapy for heart failure
- Avoid digoxin if possible
- Institute ultrafiltration or hemodialysis

■ **Pearl**

Angiotensin-converting enzyme inhibitors are central to the management of congestive heart failure due to systolic dysfunction. Modest elevations in serum creatinine (≤40% above baseline) can be tolerated as long as hyperkalemia and hypotension are avoided. If the patient's heart failure improves, the creatinine often decreases.

Reference

Marenzi G et al: Cardiac and renal dysfunction in chronic heart failure: Relation to neurohumoral activation and prognosis. Am J Med Sci 2001;321:359.

Rheumatoid Arthritis & the Heart

- Essentials of Diagnosis
  - Clinical evidence of rheumatoid arthritis
  - Pericarditis and myocarditis with characteristic granuloma on biopsy
  - Granulomatous heart valve disease, predominantly of the mitral and aortic valves

- Differential Diagnosis
  - Other causes of acute pericarditis or myocarditis
  - Other causes of valvular heart disease
  - Other connective tissue diseases

- Treatment
  - Anti-inflammatory pharmacotherapy
  - Pericardiocentesis as necessary
  - Appropriate therapy for valvular heart disease

- Pearl

The pericardial fluid is exudative and serosanquinous but has a characteristically low glucose level.

Reference

Nossent H: Risk of cardiovascular events and effect on mortality in patients with rheumatoid arthritis. J Rheumatol 2000;27:2282.

Scleroderma & the Heart

- **Essentials of Diagnosis**
  - Sclerotic skin, esophageal dysfunction, Raynaud phenomenon
  - Heart failure
  - Multisegmental myocardial perfusion abnormalities
  - Cor pulmonale

- **Differential Diagnosis**
  - Typical coronary artery disease
  - Other causes of myopericarditis and heart failure
  - Other causes of pulmonary hypertension and cor pulmonale

- **Treatment**
  - Specific anti-inflammatory pharmacotherapy
  - Calcium channel blockers for Raynaud phenomenon and pulmonary hypertension
  - Pericardiocentesis as necessary

- **Pearl**

Clinical heart failure in scleroderma is usually due to secondary involvement of the heart from systemic or pulmonary hypertension.

Reference

Murata I et al: Diversity of myocardial involvement in systemic sclerosis: An 8-year study of 9 Japanese patients. Am Heart J 1998;135:960.

Sexual Dysfunction in Cardiac Disease

■ Essentials of Diagnosis
- Erectile dysfunction is more prevalent in patients with cardio-vascular disease
- Dysfunction can be primary, or secondary to risk factors such as hypertension, diabetes, cigarette smoking, and hypercholesterolemia
- Not much is known about female sexual dysfunction in cardio-vascular disease
- Leriche syndrome and vascular impotence may occasionally cause erectile dysfunction
- Sexual intercourse increases oxygen demand by about 3–5 metabolic equivalents; any patient who is free of ischemia on submaximal exercise test can safely have vaginal intercourse

■ Differential Diagnosis
- Psychogenic impotence
- Medication-induced sexual dysfunction
- Autonomic neuropathy

■ Treatment
- Oral sildenafil is effective for erectile dysfunction (caution with concurrent nitroglycerin use)
- Give transurethral or cavernosal alprostadil (prostaglandin E1) if nitrates cannot be stopped
- Future options may include phosphodiesterase-5 inhibitors such as vardenafil and tadalafil

■ Pearl

Concurrent use of sildenafil and nitroglycerin may result in serious hypotension. Consider beta-blockers or calcium channel blockers as alternate antianginal therapy.

Reference

Solomon H et al: Relation of erectile dysfunction to angiographic coronary artery disease. Am J Cardiol 2003;91:230.

Sudden Death in Athletes

- **Essentials of Diagnosis**
  - Sudden unexplained death or cardiovascular arrest in a trained athlete is rare but receives considerable attention
  - Incidence increases with age because of concomitant coronary artery disease
  - Occurrence is unrelated to athletic performance or level of training
  - Incidence is higher if the athlete has symptoms or a family history of sudden death at a young age

- **Differential Diagnosis**
  - In athletes younger than 35, the most common underlying diseases are hypertrophic cardiomyopathy, arrhythmogenic right ventricle, congenital coronary anomalies, Marfan syndrome, congenital aortic stenosis, pre-excitation syndrome, and prolonged QT syndromes
  - In athletes older than 35 years, coronary artery disease is prevalent
  - Distinguish congenital and acquired heart disease from cardiac trauma, which can result in arrhythmias (commotio cordis), rupture of cardiac structures, or dissection of great vessels

- **Treatment**
  - The best treatment is prevention; recognize the underlying disease and restrict activities as appropriate
  - Perform history and physical examination in all athletes at least every 2 years
  - The prevalence of hypertrophic cardiomyopathy in young athletes is too low to warrant routine echocardiography
  - Any cardiovascular symptoms should prompt an evaluation
  - A family history of sudden death should prompt an evaluation

- **Pearl**

Athletes should be examined by auscultation in the upright position because this diminishes innocent systolic flow murmurs, increases the intensity of the systolic murmur of hypertrophic obstructive cardiomyopathy, and does not change the murmur of aortic stenosis.

Reference

Maron BJ et al: Recommendations for preparticipation screening and the assessment of cardiovascular disease in master athletes. Circulation 2001;103:327.

Systemic Lupus Erythematosus & the Heart

■ Essentials of Diagnosis

- Musculoskeletal and mucocutaneous manifestations of systemic lupus erythematosus
- Acute pericarditis with antinuclear antibodies detected in the pericardial fluid
- Libman-Sacks vegetations and atrioventricular valve regurgitation
- Myocarditis and vascular thrombotic disease

■ Differential Diagnosis

- Other causes of acute pericarditis or myocarditis
- Other causes of valvular heart disease
- Other causes of vascular thrombosis
- Other connective tissue diseases

■ Treatment

- Anti-inflammatory pharmacotherapy
- Pericardiocentesis as necessary
- Appropriate therapy for valvular heart disease
- Anticoagulation for thromboembolic disease

■ Pearl

Because of the high frequency of valvular lesions in systemic lupus erythematosus and their propensity to come and go, antibiotic prophylaxis for endocarditis is indicated.

Reference

Roldan CA et al: An echocardiographic study of valvular heart disease associated with systemic lupus erythematosus. N Engl J Med 1996;335:1424.

Tricyclic Antidepressants, Cardiac Effects

- ■ **Essentials of Diagnosis**
    - Properties similar to those of class I antiarrhythmic agents; also QT interval prolongation
    - Orthostatic hypotension secondary to alpha-1-adrenergic receptor blockade may cause frequent falls, particularly in the elderly
    - Ventricular proarrhythmia may occur in patients with serious structural heart disease
    - Tricyclic antidepressant overdose carries a mortality rate of 2–3% secondary to cardiac complications
    - QRS prolongation (>100 ms) is a sign of toxicity; rightward deviation of terminal 40 ms of the QRS is the most sensitive marker of toxicity (rightward terminal R wave in aVR)

- ■ **Differential Diagnosis**
    - Overdose of anticholinergic agents
    - Brugada syndrome

- ■ **Treatment (overdose)**
    - Aggressive supportive measures such as gastric lavage, airway maintenance, and activated charcoal
    - Alkalinization with IV bicarbonate for cardiac arrest, hypotension, arrhythmias, acidosis, and QRS prolongation

- ■ **Pearl**

Orthostatic hypotension is less likely to be a problem with nortriptyline than with amitriptyline or imipramine.

Reference

Witchel HJ et al: Psychotropic drugs, cardiac arrhythmia, and sudden death. J Clin Psychopharmacol 2003;23:58.

Index